M I N D F U L
PREGNANCY

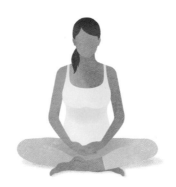

MINDFUL
PREGNANCY

MEDITATION · YOGA · HYPNOBIRTHING · NATURAL REMEDIES · NUTRITION

TRIMESTER BY TRIMESTER

TRACY DONEGAN

Registered Midwife

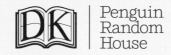

Senior Designer	Saffron Stocker
Senior Project Editor	Claire Wedderburn-Maxwell
Senior Art Editors	Emma Forge and Tom Forge
Editorial Assistant	Kiron Gill
Jacket Designer	Nicola Powling
Jacket Coordinator	Lucy Philpott
Producer, Pre-production	Heather Blagden
Senior Producer	Luca Bazzoli
Creative Technical Support	Sonia Charbonnier
Managing Editor	Dawn Henderson
Managing Art Editor	Marianne Markham
Art Director	Maxine Pedliham
Publishing Director	Mary-Clare Jerram

Illustrator	Keith Hagan
Photographer	Tara Fisher
Food Stylist	Tamara Vos
Prop Stylist	Robert Merrett

Disclaimer, see page 224

First published in Great Britain in 2020 by
Dorling Kindersley Limited
80 Strand, London, WC2R 0RL

A CIP catalogue record for this book
is available from the British Library.

ISBN: 978-0-2414-1051-6

Printed and bound in China

A WORLD OF IDEAS:
SEE ALL THERE IS TO KNOW

www.dk.com

Contents

Foreword

Pregnancy presents us with an opportunity to "come home" to our body in a way many of us haven't experienced since we were uninhibited toddlers. Mindfulness goes one step further and invites us to really feel at home in the changing landscape of our body and mind, with acceptance and appreciation for this incredible experience.

As a new mum the pressure to be perfect and look like we have it all figured out can make the transition to motherhood more difficult. Mindfulness has the potential to change our relationship with our thoughts, emotions, and with the world. It's not a magic wand, but it allows us some grace and space to approach our inner and outer world with a generous attitude of curiosity, kindness, and care. We begin to see ourselves as worthy of as much kindness and gentleness as we give to our newborn baby.

Life seems to be getting busier and more stressful, yet there is often still an unwritten expectation that mums-to-be should just keep on going while doing the most awe-inspiring job imaginable – growing a human being! Many of you reading this book are holding down full-time jobs, studying, raising a family, or looking after elderly parents. Slowing down doesn't seem to be an option. This book invites you to pause and engage in your pregnancy in a way that may initially feel foreign, but can change the way you experience your pregnancy both physically and emotionally.

My goal is to offer you a "real-world" mindfulness practice and to explore the concept of "kindfulness" (a combination of mindfulness and self-compassion). As mothers we tend to put our own needs last, but as the saying goes: "You can't pour from an empty cup." The exercises in

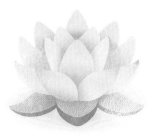

this book are not another thing to add to your already lengthy list, but a practice that you can weave into your present day-to-day life. With the avalanche of information and advice coming at you from every direction, I want to help you find a little more headspace, a little more heart space, and a lot less stress so you can focus on what really matters. Think of mindfulness as a raft that will help you feel more stable and centred in the rolling seas of change.

Your mindfulness practice will help you to stay calmer and more focused in labour as you employ mindful breathing and mindful movement, and a sense of acceptance of your experience as it is unfolding. I often hear from my midwife colleagues that many mums who have adopted a GentleBirth mindful practice don't show the usual signs of labour, such as fear and excessive pain. Calm, focused, mindful attention in labour often results in more efficient surges, and midwives are often surprised by the speed of progress.

Use the nutritional advice, exercises, and remedies in this book throughout your pregnancy, following the trimester-by-trimester approach to choose what feels right for you as your pregnancy progresses. Practise the yoga sequences to promote calmness, strength, and flexibility each trimester, as they are adapted to suit your changing body and to get you ready, both mentally and physically, for birth.

The benefits of mindfulness are cumulative, and adopting the practices that resonate most with you will help you to have the healthiest, most enjoyable pregnancy possible, a more positive and empowered birth, and the headspace to embrace your new role as a mother. "All is well."

Tracy Donegan

A MINDFUL PREGNANCY

Pregnancy is a time of complex changes and growth, yet some of the most profound changes are the ones you can't see. Your inner world of emotions shifts constantly, but approaching your pregnancy in a mindful way will benefit both you and your baby as your thoughts and emotions flourish with more ease and less anxiety.

What is a mindful pregnancy?

Mindfulness will nourish and nurture you as you learn to pay attention to your current experience. It will allow you to fully connect with your heart, mind, body, and baby on the incredible journey of pregnancy.

Having a mindful approach to your pregnancy means learning how to stay present – in the moment as it unfolds. You are training your mind to let go of any worries or negative thoughts that come and go so you can enjoy your pregnancy with minimal stress. It can also help you become more accepting of your feelings about pregnancy and birth, especially if you're not enjoying some parts of your pregnancy as much as you think you "should be".

As you become more mindful while doing simple daily activities such as taking a shower *(see p60)* or eating *(see p84)*, your mind will wander less to worrying about future events; or replaying bad decisions from the past.

Mindfulness is all about focus – and where you put that focus will have a profound influence on how much you enjoy this season in your life. Focus is like a muscle that gets stronger: the more you practise being mindful, the easier you will adapt to the intensity of emotions that come with the changes of becoming a new mum.

All of the practices in this book support emotional and physical wellness throughout your pregnancy and as you adapt to being a parent. With daily practice, a mindful approach to pregnancy can be life-changing. What better time to feel calm, confident, and in control than as you prepare to meet your baby?

A MINDFUL FRAMEWORK FOR PREGNANCY

These interconnected mindful "pillars" can transform your pregnancy as you attend to your thoughts and feelings. At different times you may find you're drawn to different pillars.

Beginner's mind

Look at the world as if this is the first time you hear, see, or feel something – just like your baby experiencing life for the first time.

Gratitude

When you give thanks for all the goodness in your pregnancy, you will find it is hard to be in a bad mood and grateful at the same time.

Acceptance

Memorize these four words: 'This too shall pass". If everything is constantly changing, then it's easier to tolerate a low patch.

Letting go

Notice your judging in an easy-going way with a curious attitude; and let go of unrealistic expectations you have of yourself and others.

Patience

Parenting requires unlimited patience – with yourself and your baby, so allow yourself the time and grace to appreciate your feelings.

Trust

Trust your "gut" when it comes to pregnancy. Practise the exercises in this book to help you appreciate your natural instincts.

"Have an 'open door' policy to all of your feelings during pregnancy."

The pregnant mind

You may well have experienced the symptoms of "baby brain", such as putting your car keys in the fridge. During pregnancy, profound changes are occurring in your brain as parts of it are remodelled for motherhood.

It's no secret that hormones influence how your brain works in pregnancy, and parts of your brain become extra "plastic" so that you will bond and respond to your newborn baby instinctively. However, when you focus on curating positive thoughts and emotions, your mindful approach can change your brain in many positive ways. Just as important is the fact that your emotional state can shape your baby's brain, too.

A mindful approach to pregnancy invites you to simply be an observer of your scattered thoughts so your baby basks in "happy hormones", and you react in a more balanced way to the unpredictabilities of pregnancy.

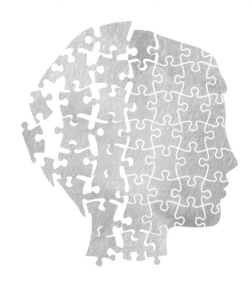

EASY MINDFUL PRACTICES FOR PREGNANCY

Follow these simple mindfulness tips every day so that you feel calmer, more focused, more relaxed, and less stressed throughout your pregnancy and into motherhood.

Be grateful

As soon as you wake up, and before your brain starts worrying, take a moment to appreciate someone or something in your life.

Brush your teeth mindfully

Pay attention to how your body feels: how your jaw moves, and how your toothpaste tastes.

Befriend your emotions

Don't categorize feelings or thoughts into "good" or "bad". Acknowledge their presence and allow them to simply pass.

Eat mindfully

Eat slowly, taste your food properly, and breathe in the aroma, so you mindfully enjoy your meal. *See also p24 and p84.*

Pay attention to your breathing

During your commute or while doing the shopping, focus on your breathing. Is it deep or shallow? *See also p16.*

Slow down

Look at what is all around you. Take a mindful walk (*see p64*) and notice the trees, the bird song, and the temperature of the air.

Redirect your focus

If you feel anxious, simply redirect your focus out of your head and into your body by focusing on your feet.

Connect with your baby

Imagine holding your baby, counting her tiny toes, seeing her first steps, and hearing her first spoken words.

Be your best friend

Speak to yourself kindly, and treat your pregnant body gently. You are growing a human being – how amazing is that!

Meditation

The nurturing practice of meditation will support you throughout your pregnancy. Even short meditations promote emotional positivity and stability as well as having a calming effect on your body and baby.

As humans we have what's known as "monkey" or "puppy" brain. It jumps from thought to thought, emotion to emotion, has a very short attention span, and gets caught up in the drama of our inner experience.

Meditation helps to train your mind for a more enjoyable, less stressful pregnancy and labour. It doesn't magically turn you into a pregnant Zen master overnight. It just helps you to step back and see what's happening from a broader perspective.

Think of meditation as an umbrella term for different types of mental focus, including deliberately sitting or intentionally moving in a mindful way, for example doing yoga or t'ai chi.

Importance of meditation

When you are feeling stressed or overwhelmed, you just don't have the headspace to see past your fear, anger, or disappointment, and the part of your brain associated with making rational decisions is offline. Meditation calms the emotional part of your mind, allowing you to see more clearly.

Pregnancy brings with it lots of important decisions and you want to make those decisions from a place of calm and wise intention – when was the last time you made a good decision in a bad mood?

Recent research also suggests that meditation is excellent for navigating the waves of sensations in labour by increasing your mental focus, which reduces pain.

Is it safe?

Meditation is considered safe for pregnancy, but if at any point you find any of the exercises uncomfortable, stop and make sure you consult with your health-care provider.

"Meditate every day to tune into your inner wisdom and compassion for yourself and your baby."

BENEFITS OF MEDITATION

The more mindful you are during your pregnancy, the more you and your baby get to experience the cumulative benefits of meditation. Below are some of the many advantages:

Better sleep

Enjoy improved sleep quality, and even if sleep deprived you're more likely to have improved day-to-day brain functioning.

Good connections

You will experience a deeper bond with your unborn baby. Your relationship with your partner will also be enriched.

Enhanced mood

You're likely to feel more positive and meditating may reduce your risk of postnatal depression and/or anxiety.

Healthy weight

You are more likely to have a healthy weight gain during pregnancy; and your baby is more likely to be within a normal weight range.

Stress reduction

You'll feel less reactive to stress and more emotionally resilient. Many women report feeling less fear and pain in labour.

Reduced risks

Your baby is less likely to be born prematurely and is more likely to experience healthy brain functioning due to your reduced stress.

Mindful breathing

Bringing all of your attention to your breath will make you feel more in control and less reactive to stress and worry during pregnancy. It will also prove invaluable during labour to help you stay focused and energized.

Focusing mindfully on your breath is the practice of simply noticing your inhale and exhale at various times throughout your day. It helps to calm the "puppy" brain and is one of the most effective ways to cope with negative thoughts or experiences. It can help with emotional stability throughout pregnancy as it soothes powerful emotions.

Many of us shallow breathe (only breathing into the rib cage), but deep, satisfying belly breathing (like all newborns do) is more beneficial.

When you breathe in, it speeds up your heart rate, so if you lengthen the out breath just a little you're maximizing your relaxation response. Imagine any tension in your body just melting away with that out breath.

Mindful breathing allows you to gently pause the non-stop chatter of a busy pregnant mind while intentionally increasing oxygen to your body and growing baby. A few mindful breaths can become an instant soothing sanctuary within which your mind, body, and baby are connected.

"Connect to inner calm through your breath during pregnancy and on the day you meet your baby."

Breathing mindfully throughout your pregnancy will also ensure you have a good foundation in place for labour.

Breathing during labour

As your pregnancy progresses, you will probably read articles about breathing techniques, but there's no secret to how to breathe during labour. That's because your body just adapts to the activity. In early labour you'll breathe normally. As you enter the active labour phase you'll find you need to pause during a surge and breathe deeply. Concentrate on slow, focused breathing, which will relax you and give you increased stamina, and just let your body do the work naturally.

If you're overly anxious in labour, mindful breathing can reduce feelings of panic as surges move through your body, which can feel overwhelming. Focusing on your breathing will help you stay calm and more in control.

Is it safe?

Mindful breathing is completely safe. However, if at any time it feels uncomfortable, stop and consult your health-care provider.

Pregnancy yoga

Yoga brings together a combination of gentle exercises, mindfulness, relaxation, and breathing techniques. It is the ideal way to connect your mind, body, breath, and baby during all the stages of pregnancy and labour.

The yoga poses and exercises in this book can help with flexibility, strength, and focus. They have been been adapted for each trimester so you can tailor them to your stage of pregnancy.

If you've been used to high-intensity exercise before you became pregnant, yoga can seem a little unsatisfying in the beginning, but stick with it.

As with any type of exercise, there are a few things to be aware of. Use a yoga mat to avoid slipping, and, as your pregnancy progresses, use blocks, cushions, or blankets to provide extra support where needed. Avoid poses that involve lying flat on your back after 18 weeks, and stop straight away if any pose is painful or makes you feel dizzy or nauseous.

Is it safe?
Gentle yoga is safe to practise throughout your pregnancy, but note that this is not a time to be pushing your body. If you have any concerns, talk to your health-care provider.

"Antenatal yoga is all about calmness, comfort, connection, and confidence."

BENEFITS OF YOGA DURING PREGNANCY

Yoga can help you to embrace your pregnancy by calming your mind and strengthening your body, as well as preparing you mentally and physically for labour.

Focused breathing

One very important aspect of antenatal yoga is mindful breathing *(see p16)*. Simple, focused breathing exercises will calm your body and your mind.

Build flexibility, strength, and stamina

Squats *(see p107* and *p146)* are great for your legs, lower back, and pelvic floor, and it's something that will feel really productive in active labour *(see p184* and *p188)*. Low Lunges *(see p145)* build flexibility in your hips and strength in your legs. Exercises that open the hips, such as Squats *(see p107* and *p146)*, Butterfly *(see p154),* and Pigeon Poses *(see pp112–3* and *p152)* are essential to make room for your baby and encourage your baby into the optimal position for birth.

Relieve aches

Yoga can help with backache, headaches, and normal pregnancy swelling. Cat and Cow *(see p109* and *p148)* can ease backache; while the relaxing Resting Pose *(see p75, p115,* and *p157)* can relieve headaches.

Take time for yourself

Practising yoga every day *(see p68, p100, p142,* and *p214* for sequences)* will help to keep you calm, and give you time to focus on enjoying your pregnancy and bonding with your baby.

Sense of community

An enjoyable aspect of antenatal yoga is the sense of community if you join a class, finding a supportive group of fellow mums-to-be to share tips and reassurance.

Natural remedies

Many expectant mums are keen to find safe, natural ways to reduce pregnancy discomforts. Exploring natural remedies doesn't mean turning your back on medicine, just being more mindful about your care.

All these natural remedies are safe to use in pregnancy (some you may wish to try after the first trimester), but check with your midwife first.

You may find some remedies are more effective than others, and there may be some pregnancy discomforts or challenges that you can't alleviate with natural or even medical options. Something that might have been considered an old wives' tale can make the difference between an enjoyable pregnancy and a challenging one. Cultivating a holistic, mindful approach to pregnancy can also help you feel more in control of your wellbeing and your baby's. A guiding principle of mindfulness is that nothing stays the same and it's very likely that some of these discomforts will pass.

Quelling nausea

For many newly expectant mums experiencing "normal" morning sickness, ginger is usually the first remedy they try. It can be taken many ways – as a tea, candied, as a supplement, or in a food *(see p53)*.

Other helpful holistic remedies for a queasy tummy include the use of essential oils, especially citrus and peppermint oils *(see p54)*.

"A mindful approach to pregnancy can help you feel more in control."

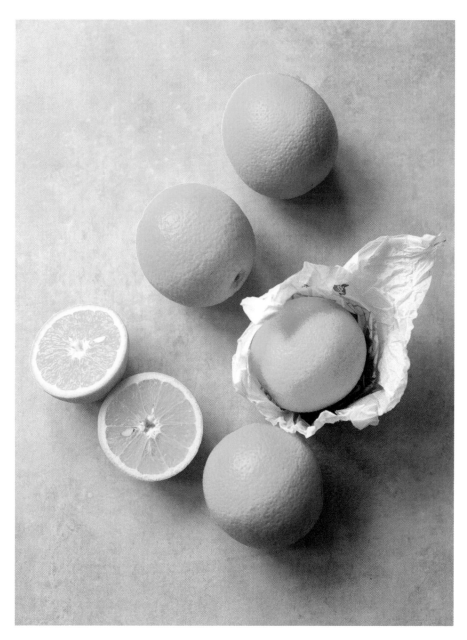

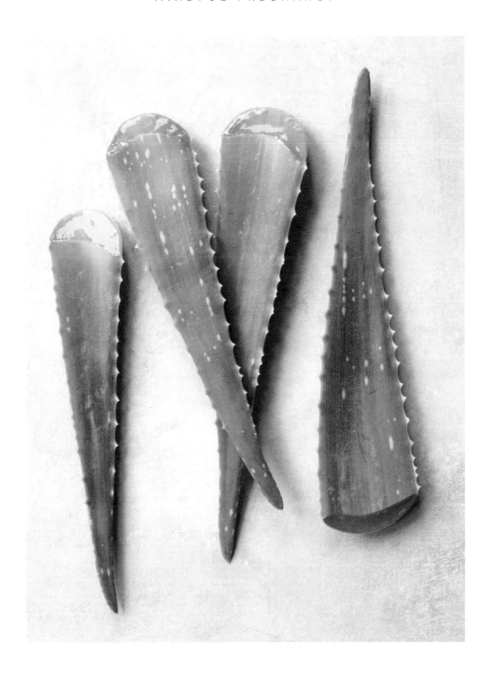

Calming remedies

It's totally normal that some mums will experience anxiety and worry during pregnancy. Most anxiety is caused by our thoughts, which often focus on what can go wrong during pregnancy and birth rather than what usually goes right. Remedies for anxiety include the well-known Bach Rescue Remedy and Mimulus Flower remedy.

Improved sleep

Many women experience disrupted sleep during pregnancy. Essential oils such as lavender or chamomile *(see p98)*, massages, and warm baths are all considered safe, natural aids to help sleep quality after the first trimester.

Soothing remedies

Cold packs, herbal baths *(see p212)*, and cool witch hazel can all reduce the swelling associated with haemorrhoids, a common pregnancy complaint.

Healthy skin

Stretch marks tend to appear during times of rapid growth and weight gain. As the skin stretches it can cause uncomfortable itching on the thighs and belly, but there are ways to minimize this. Beef bone broth contains collagen that improves skin elasticity, and is also a great option if you have morning sickness.

Make moisturizing a nourishing ritual and connect lovingly with your body. Apply a natural moisturizer, such as aloe vera, daily. Start with your feet and work your way up, including your belly *(see p90)*.

Optimal perineal care

Research suggests that perineal massage *(see p130)* in the last few weeks of pregnancy may reduce perineal injury. After the birth, to ease any discomfort you can make your own soothing padsicles *(see p212)*. A couple of days postpartum you can begin having warm, herbal baths *(see p212)* to soothe and promote perineal healing.

Encouraging milk supply

The first few days of breastfeeding bring about noticeable changes to your breasts, including engorgement. Cool, soothing cabbage leaves on your breasts can reduce discomfort *(see p200)*.

There are also a number of herbal remedies, such as fenugreek, that can help if you are experiencing low milk supply *(see p205)*.

Nutrition

Eating well is one of the most important aspects of "building" a baby, and you can reduce the likelihood of future complications by being mindful of what you eat, how you eat, and by choosing a well-balanced diet.

You are creating a human being, so you want to use the best "materials" possible. Pregnancy can be stressful and unless you have the skills to manage the rollercoaster of emotions you are more likely to eat mindlessly, which means you may choose less healthy foods or overeat.

Eating mindfully means that you won't rush your food, but instead will taste the food properly, taking time to enjoy your food when you are hungry. It can help you become more aware of when you are actually hungry (rather than bored or stressed, for example) and when you are full. You will start to understand how emotions impact hunger, and learn to savour your food.

Stress is a trigger for overeating as your body produces more stress hormones signalling your brain to drive you to consume more high-calorie foods. Eating mindfully and thinking about how your baby benefits from your diet can help you to make good nutritious choices – so, rather than reaching for a quick-fix biscuit, have a handful of walnuts, which are a great source of omega-3 fatty acids (*see p82*); or try snacking on sunflower seeds, which are rich in vitamin B (*see p48*).

Benefits for your baby

For most expectant mums nothing is more important than having a healthy baby, and we know without a doubt that how you nourish your body in pregnancy can reduce your likelihood of experiencing complications and can set your baby's trajectory for a lifetime of optimal health and wellbeing. Your daily food choices will influence your pregnancy, your birth, and your newborn's long-term health.

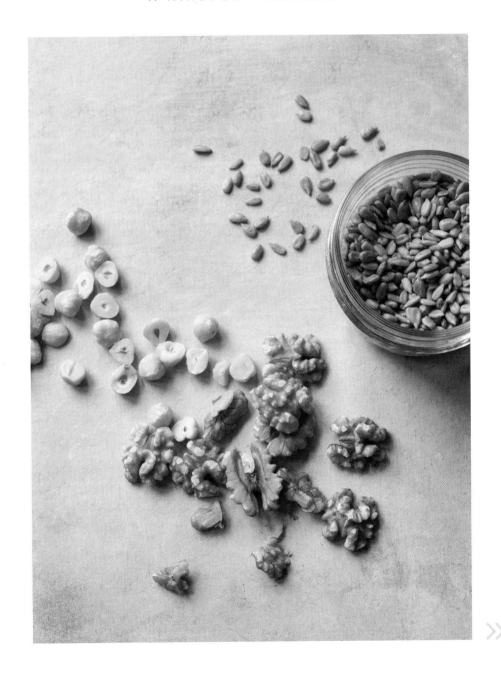

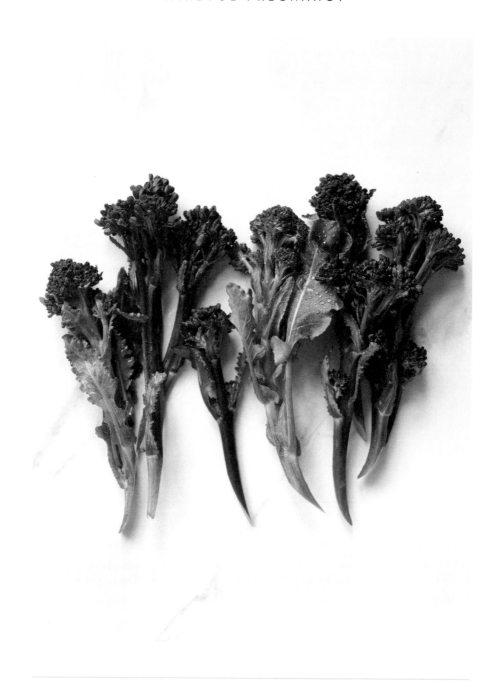

You are what you eat

You may believe that you have a reasonably healthy diet, but research suggests that a large percentage of expectant mothers are deficient in key nutrients. Make sure you enjoy a good selection of colourful fruit and vegetables, such as broccoli, sweet potatoes, and berries; pulses and lentils; as well as eggs; lean meat and white fish.

For a healthy, balanced diet in pregnancy you need good sources of protein *(see p67)*; "good fats" *(see p82)*; fibre *(see p94)*; and carbohydrates. Try to eat unprocessed complex carbohydrates as they give you energy for longer. For example, choose wholegrain bread or brown rice rather than refined white bread or white rice.

You also need a number of important minerals and vitamins including calcium *(see p45)*; Vitamin D *(see p62)*; B vitamins *(see p48)*; iodine and choline *(see p59)*; folate *(see p40)*; and zinc, a mineral that helps with many functions including foetal cell division and growth. In addition, drink plenty of water to stay well hydrated.

If you are vegetarian or vegan you may need to take extra care with balancing your diet to gain all the nutrients your baby needs, so talk to your health-care provider about ways to ensure you have the optimal diet.

HUNGER MEDITATION

You may find it best to eat regular, small meals when pregnant, but if you are simply craving snacks, try this meditation first.

1 Take three deep, slow breaths and ask yourself – am I really feeling hungry or am I just bored, lonely, or stressed? Not sure? Drink a glass of water first. **2** If you are hungry, try to choose a healthy option and savour it – noting the texture and taste of your food. **3** If you are craving an unhealthy treat, think: "Will eating this contribute to having a healthy pregnancy?" **4** If you do have the treat, eat it mindfully without judgment, and then repeat the above steps if another craving starts.

≫

Eating for two?

There is still a strong belief that when you are pregnant you can eat for two. However, scientists now suggest you should "eat for 1.1", choosing healthy fresh foods and cutting out processed foods whenever possible.

Pregnant women only need 200–300 additional calories in pregnancy starting in the second trimester. The trick is to make your calories count instead of counting the calories; finding foods that are packed with vitamins and minerals that will nourish both you and your baby.

Eating a balanced diet may help you to avoid problems during pregnancy such as gestational diabetes, premature birth, and anaemia. If you have a high BMI, then this is not the time to diet, but take steps to have the healthiest pregnancy possible. No matter what your body type is, or how fit you are, try to appreciate how good nutrition can benefit you during pregnancy.

Foods to avoid

The NHS recommends that pregnant women do not eat pâté, liver, raw or undercooked meats, raw shellfish, shark, swordfish, or marlin, and more than two portions a week of oily fish. It's also advised not to eat uncooked mould-ripened soft cheeses, such as brie or camembert, or soft blue-veined cheeses, such as gorgonzola or roquefort, unless cooked thoroughly.

Eggs not produced under the British Lion Code of Practice (stamped with a logo) should be thoroughly cooked to prevent the risk of salmonella.

Check with your health-care provider for a full list of what is safe to eat or what to avoid while pregnant.

"Choose nutrient-dense foods such as dried beans, which are also good sources of protein and fibre."

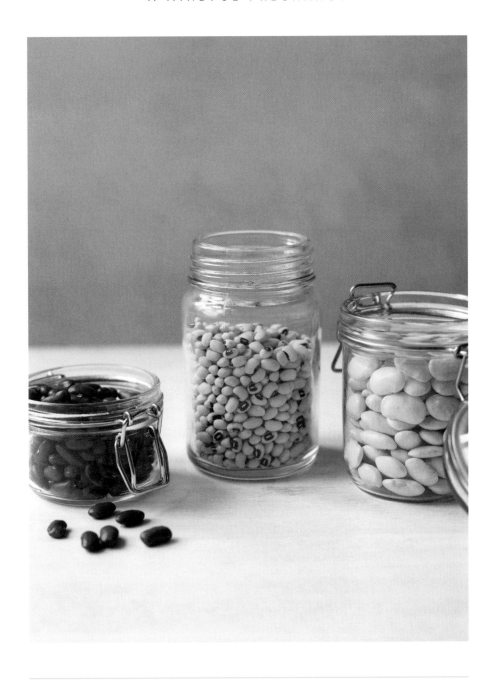

Hypnobirthing

This specialist birth preparation programme has grown in popularity around the world. It aims to retrain your brain so that you have a more relaxed, more comfortable, and more confident pregnancy and labour.

Hypnobirthing teaches breathing, relaxation, and self-hypnosis techniques so you can have an empowered pregnancy and birth.

By practising hypnobirthing throughout your pregnancy you can help to alleviate some common pregnancy discomforts, such as morning sickness, as well as connecting fully with your baby in the early trimesters as you start your journey to becoming a new mother.

Later, during your labour and birth you can use hypnosis techniques to stay focused and reduce stress, helping you to have a positive birth experience. For some women hypnobirthing may help to reduce pain in labour, although note that it does not guarantee a pain-free labour.

There are so many myths around hypnosis, but at no time when hypnobirthing are you "under a spell",

in a trance, under the control of anyone other than yourself, or able to get "stuck". You are totally in control, fully awake, and aware of everything that's going on around you.

Hypnobirthing in pregnancy

Hypnobirthing is an effective tool to use throughout your pregnancy to improve sleep quality, reduce nausea *(see p50)*, lower stress, and soothe some physical discomforts as your pregnancy progresses. Choose imagery that feels good and lifts your emotions as it will be the most effective.

Hypnobirthing techniques will also give you more confidence in your ability to have a gentle, positive birth and feel less worried about labour in the lead-up to the birth. Indeed, many mums start to feel more excited about their baby's birth within a few days of starting hypnobirthing exercises.

"Every mother deserves to enjoy a positive pregnancy and birth."

BENEFITS OF HYPNOBIRTHING

Research shows that regularly practising hypnobirthing exercises can bring many benefits to both you and your baby, not just during labour but throughout your pregnancy.

Relieves symptoms

You can use hypnobirthing techniques from the first trimester to help relieve symptoms of morning sickness and fatigue.

Reduced risk of complications

You are less likely to have complications during labour due to your reduced stress levels.

Increased focus during labour

You may find labour seems to pass more quickly and you can stay focused throughout as your stress and pain levels are lower.

Reduction in pain

You may not require medication. Many mums report their labour sensations are intense but not excruciatingly painful.

Calmer baby

Your baby may be healthier and calmer as a more relaxed mum equals a more relaxed baby.

Improved outcome

If you have a caesarean, then research suggests that you may spend less time in surgery and need less pain medication afterwards.

"Mums who use imagery during labour consistently report feeling more relaxed and in control."

BIRTH VISION BOARD

During your pregnancy, make a collection of inspiring, calming, and confidence-building images and quotes to remind you that birth can be a beautiful experience.

Get into the zone

You can make a vision board on your own or with a group of expectant mums. If you're doing it alone it can be a lovely meditative practice. Take your time, light a candle or put on relaxing music, and settle down with a selection of magazines.

Create the feeling

Find images, affirmations, and quotes that resonate strongly with you – the most important thing is not how pretty the images are, but how they make you feel. When you look at the board you should be inspired and reassured.

Reinforce the vision

Visualization is a powerful hypnobirthing tool to prepare for a mindful birth. Creating a sacred space focused on positive images of birth and placing it in your home where you'll see it frequently is like doing lots of mini visualizations every day. Also take it with you to your place of birth so you can reconnect with those feelings of confidence and inspiration.

Hypnobirthing in labour

Most of us have already been "hypnotized" to believe that labour involves long, frightening hours of agonizing stress and pain. It is something to just "get through". Women haven't lost the ability to give birth instinctively, but in this world of constant distraction and stress, many parents have lost the ability to intentionally remain calm during physically and mentally demanding challenges such as labour and birth.

Hypnobirthing retrains your brain so that you expect your baby's birth will be an empowering experience rather than a traumatic one. It is an "off switch" for adrenaline, which is a chemical messenger that kicks in when you are afraid, tightens your muscles, and is known to make labour longer and more painful. Without the presence of adrenaline caused by fear and anxiety your body is naturally filled with endorphins and oxytocin – you make your own epidural and natural pain-relievers.

It is worth watching a video of mothers using hypnobirthing techniques, as they are awake, alert, incredibly focused, and even joking between surges. In fact, these inspiring videos are almost strange to watch as we're just not used to seeing birth as such a positive, quiet, calm, and uplifting experience.

You will always be aware of what is happening to you and around you, and never detached from the experience, which is a common misconception.

How do I do it?

Practise the hypnobirthing exercises in this book regularly. In addition, use an app *(see p224)* or CD, which you may find more relaxing, or take a class. When practising the exercises, allow your mind to drift off into relaxation. You may not hear all of the content, but as long as your stress levels reduce over the weeks, you're doing it right.

If you do want to find a class, get advice from other mothers and choose carefully so you find one that will help you to have the best pregnancy and labour experience possible.

Is it safe?

Hypnobirthing is considered a safe practice during pregnancy, but if you find any of the exercises bring up difficult emotions stop and talk to your health-care provider.

Also, do not use the techniques while driving or at any time when your attention is required elsewhere.

YOUR FIRST TRIMESTER

Your body is starting its amazing transformation so that your baby can flourish in optimal conditions. Here we'll explore ways to nourish yourself emotionally, physically, and nutritionally during the important first 12 weeks. You'll also find suggestions for natural remedies to increase your comfort in this trimester.

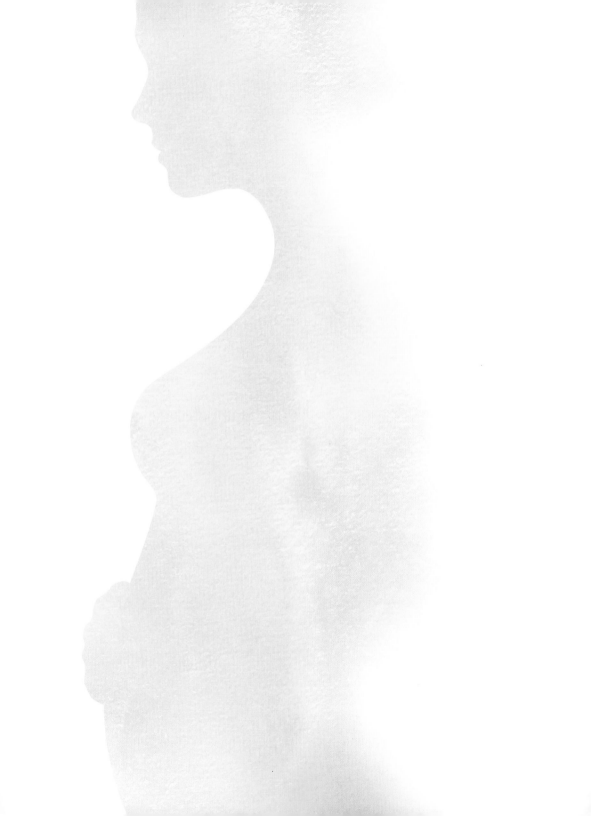

What's happening?

Although you won't have a bump yet, this is a time of incredible adaptations – all happening behind the scenes. Every system of your body is altering to provide the healthiest environment for your baby.

Many of these changes are happening as early as 8–10 weeks into your pregnancy, before you even have your first antenatal visit. Not only is your body transforming – so is your identity. You are embarking on the biggest transition of your adult life. With all these physical and emotional changes, it's not surprising most newly expectant mums experience fatigue and mood swings in the first trimester.

As your body goes through a major transformation in the first 12 weeks you may find that you have sore or sensitive breasts. Those hard-working hormones can also trigger morning sickness *(see p50, p53, and p54 for ways to help with this).*

Your digestive system is starting to slow down as your body retrieves nutrients from your diet to grow your baby, making it even more important to

"Be gentle with yourself during the first few months of pregnancy."

have a healthy and varied diet with plenty of fibre (*see p94*) to avoid constipation. You may experience bloating, and, although your kidneys are adapting to pregnancy, you are likely to have to urinate more often.

Already, your blood volume is starting to increase (it'll have almost doubled by the end of your pregnancy), and amazing changes are happening to your cardiovascular system, as your heart actually enlarges.

With all this happening, make sure that if you have been prescribed any medication pre-pregnancy, you consult with your health-care professional.

All about you

Whether this is a much longed-for pregnancy or a surprise, the emotions of the first few weeks of pregnancy can be a rollercoaster of highs and lows – excitement and disbelief, as well as anxiety and exhilaration.

A mindful approach to your emotional wellbeing and the physical changes during this time can help you to "surf" some of the more challenging emotions that you may experience, rather than feeling overwhelmed by them. Short meditations and mindful breathing can help you to feel more at ease during this trimester.

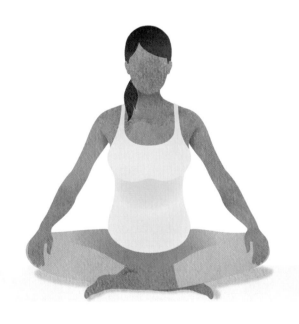

It's hard not to worry about miscarriage during the first trimester. In the vast majority of cases there is little anyone can do to prevent a miscarriage – although that doesn't take the pain away when it happens to you.

You may also worry how a new baby will impact on your body, your career, your finances, or your relationship with your partner. These feelings are normal and the sooner you can allow yourself the space and grace to approach strong emotions with curiosity and acceptance the better you'll feel. Don't worry about things you can't change – instead follow the mantra: "control the controllables".

If you're keeping your pregnancy under wraps until the second trimester, make sure you confide in a trusted friend about how you're feeling (preferably someone who has been through pregnancy already).

Pregnancy affords you a timely opportunity to reflect on your approach to life, work, and family in a way that adds a wonderful richness to your life. Always be gentle with yourself, though, and embrace "kindfulness" *(see p6)*. If you are finding the emotions of the first trimester challenging, talk to your health-care provider – not everyone finds pregnancy easy.

All about your baby

When you think about it, what's going on in your body is truly magical. In only 40 weeks the natural intelligence of your body will be able to grow a human being from just one microscopic cell.

Your baby is on a developmental fast track, and by the end of the first trimester he has gone from resembling a tadpole to a fully formed little person, about 7.5cm in length.

" A mindful pregnancy allows you to connect with the innate wisdom of your body, heart, and mind."

YOUR BABY'S DEVELOPMENT

Isn't it incredible that you can grow another human from a single cell with no conscious effort? The growth of your baby in the first trimester really is amazing.

Neural development

Your baby's brain begins to form by five weeks, before you even know you are pregnant, and will be growing at a rate of a quarter of a million cells per minute by the end of the first trimester. The spinal cord also starts to develop from the neural tube in this trimester.

Milk teeth form

Tooth buds, which will become milk teeth, are growing in the gums. By the end of this trimester your baby can open and close his mouth.

Major body systems

By the end of eight weeks all your baby's body systems are developing.

Limb formation

Your baby's arms and legs have grown from tiny nubs to being fully formed by the end of the first trimester.

Nail growth

By 12 weeks your baby will have developed tiny fingernails and toenails.

Sexual organs

By the end of the first trimester your baby's genitals will have developed.

Taste buds

Your baby's sense of taste is starting to develop as he swallows amniotic fluid flavoured with foods you've eaten.

Head size

Your baby's head makes up about half of his total body length by the end of the first trimester.

Folate and folic acid

Folate is a B vitamin that is found naturally in foods, whereas folic acid is a synthetic supplement. When possible, choose a supplement including the words "-folate" as the healthier, more natural option.

Getting enough folate or folic acid is vital for your baby's development in early pregnancy as it protects against major birth defects of the brain and spine. As it can be difficult to get the required amount of folate from your diet alone, it is recommended that anyone planning a pregnancy should take a folate or folic acid supplement for three months before conception and until the end of the first trimester. Folic acid supplements are not advised after the first trimester, but eating folate-rich foods throughout is recommended.

Good sources of folate include vegetables such as **asparagus**, **broccoli**, **beetroot**, and **cauliflower**, as well as **citrus fruits**, **lentils**, and **eggs**. Try adding an extra leafy green vegetable to your main meal to boost your folate levels – **Brussels sprouts**, **romaine lettuce**, **mustard greens**, **kale**, and **spinach** are all high in folate. Or add **kidney beans** or lentils to casseroles or soups to increase folate levels. Choose organically grown produce when possible.

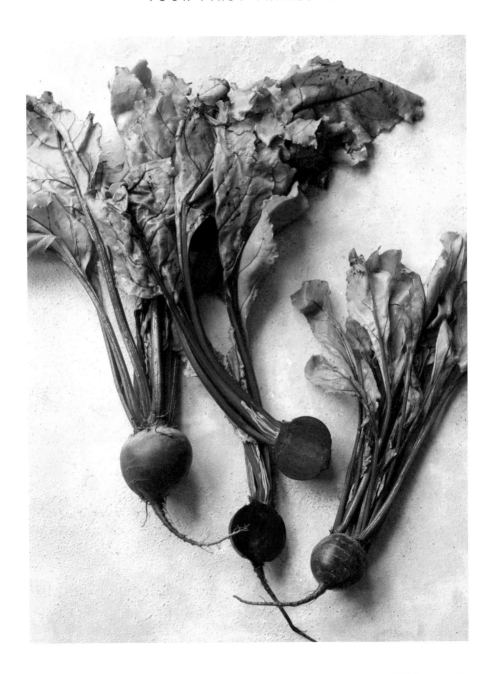

One-minute meditation

In pregnancy it's normal to worry, but focusing on those worries makes them larger than life. Practise this meditation several times a day, allowing any anxious thoughts to pass like clouds in a blue sky.

1

Sit comfortably on a chair with your feet on the ground. Close your eyes or find a spot in front of you to focus on with a soft gaze. Remember, no matter how short or long your meditation, always approach it with a warm, positive attitude.

2

As you breathe in, feel the gentle expansion of your body. As you breathe out, notice your body softening and letting go.

3

As you breathe in, notice the feeling of fullness. As you breathe out, notice the feeling of release.

4

If your mind wanders off to a thought or sensation, celebrate that moment of mindful awareness with compassion and curiosity, then gently guide your attention back to your breath. Continue this breath awareness for just one minute.

"As you become more confident and comfortable meditating, you can increase the time you meditate for."

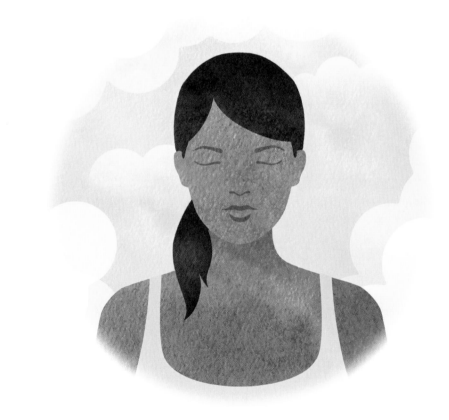

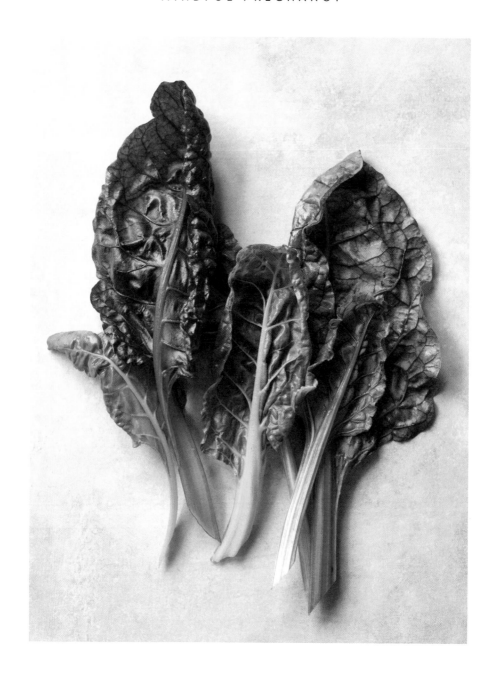

Calcium

Use a mindful approach when selecting your sources of calcium so you're intentionally choosing options that are not only rich in calcium, but provide you and your baby with other key nutrients during your pregnancy.

Calcium is vital for the growth of your baby's bones and teeth, as little tooth "buds" form in the gums during pregnancy. It is also essential for the development of your baby's muscles and heart. As your baby will take the calcium she needs from your body, making sure you have enough calcium for both of you is important. **Milk** and other **dairy products** are good sources of calcium, as are some **green leafy vegetables**.

Seeds are rich in calcium, so why not sprinkle some roasted **sesame seeds** over a **rocket** salad or steamed **Swiss chard** or **broccoli**? To boost your calcium intake, enjoy a **yoghurt** for breakfast, have a handful of **almonds** as a quick snack, or add **sardines** in olive oil to a salad for a nutritious lunch. If dairy products aren't an option for you, talk to your health-care provider about a calcium supplement.

Heart-centred breathing

During pregnancy, feelings can become overwhelming. This is an excellent technique to use whenever any challenging feelings arise, as you can do it anywhere and it will immediately help you to refocus emotionally.

1

If you feel anxious, either sit or stand and take a few slow, deep breaths. Ideally close your eyes, but you can keep them open.

2

Focus your attention on the centre of your ribs, around your heart. Breathe deeply. Imagine that your breath is moving in and out through the area of your heart. As you inhale and exhale, think of a beautiful place – a tropical rainforest, a wildflower meadow, or an Alpine mountain range.

3

As you breathe in and out, activate positive feelings such as appreciation or love. Recall a wonderful memory or special person – a grandmother who adored you unconditionally, or someone who made you feel really loved. Allow that feeling to grow and as it grows, notice how your stress decreases.

4

Finish the exercise, appreciating that by focusing on breathing and positive thoughts you can turn off the stress response.

"This technique allows you to make a powerful emotional shift within moments, bringing about balance."

Vitamin B12

Your energy levels can take a dive in pregnancy, especially in the first trimester. Vitamin B12 can boost your energy and most likely your mood, too, as it can help reduce the effects of stress.

Vitamin B12 is essential for your baby's brain development right from conception. It is involved in the metabolization of proteins, carbohydrates, and fats in your diet so your baby gets everything she needs to grow. It is also important for a healthy nervous system and works with folate/folic acid to reduce the risk of neural tube defects. If you are vegetarian or vegan you're more likely to have low B12 levels so make sure you discuss this with your health-care provider.

Good sources of vitamin B12 include **meat** (grass-fed whenever possible), **wild salmon**, **milk**, and other **dairy products** (many are fortified), **eggs**, and fortified **cereals**. Start your day with breakfast cereal with added B12 and fortified milk. Enjoy poached eggs with **ham** or **spinach** for lunch, grilled salmon for dinner, or try **yeast extract** and **cheese** on **wholemeal crackers** for a B12-rich snack.

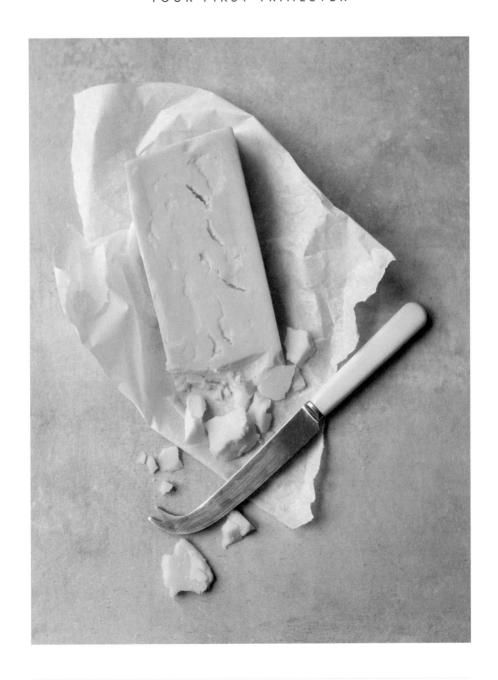

Morning wellness

Morning sickness is quite common, particularly in the first trimester. Use this exercise whenever you feel queasy to create new associations for wellness and to make your early pregnancy more comfortable.

1

Find somewhere you won't be disturbed. Follow these steps or ask your partner to read the visualization out loud to you.

2

Close your eyes. Breathe slowly in … and slowly out … at a comfortable pace for you. Notice the tension in your chest as you take a deep breath in, and as you exhale notice how that tension releases. Let your body settle as you take time to connect with the inner wisdom and wellness of your body.

3

Count from 10 down to 1, allowing each number to increasingly relax you.

10 Connect with your inner source of wisdom and wellness. **9** Release.
8 Drift and float. **7** Release even more as you easily count down. **6** Let go.
5 Relax. **4** This is your special time. **3** Double your relaxation.
2 Deepen your relaxation – then go deeper still, all the way down to
1 With practice, you should now be in a hypnotic state.

4

Imagine a very special farmer's market on a spring day. The air is cool and comfortable. You walk past colourful stalls overflowing with fresh, delicious produce. The smell of lemons and oranges fills the air. Think of a time when you were cutting ripe, juicy oranges at home and of the tanginess of fresh lemon juice. Imagine breathing in the scent of those juicy, zesty oranges or lemons, feeling healthy, breathing in wellness and vitality.

5

Count up slowly from 1 to 5 and you'll find you feel energized.

1 Breathe in those scents of wellness and vitality. **2** Breathe out any feelings of nausea. **3** Start to move your hands and feet. **4** Open your eyes. **5** Notice how good you feel.

To continue the benefits of the hypnosis, keep citrus scents around you at home or at work to immediately energize you and increase feelings of wellness.

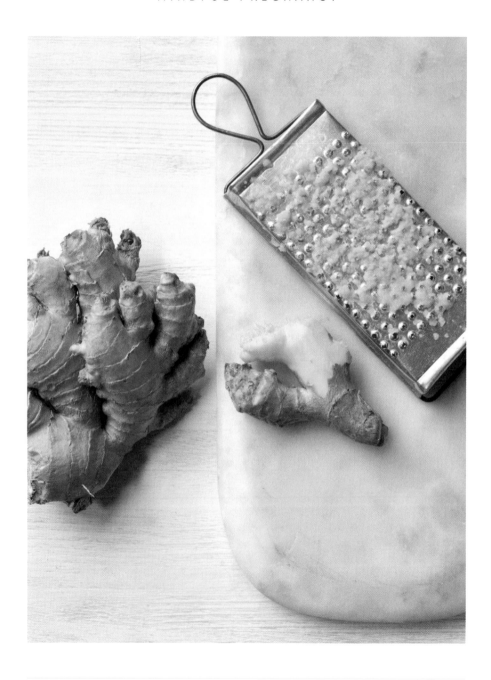

Ginger for nausea

If you're feeling nauseous due to hormonal changes in early pregnancy, ginger is one of the best-known and most effective natural remedies. Plus, it can help to alleviate common digestive problems such as bloating.

Several studies suggest **ginger** is a safe and effective way to reduce nausea and vomiting without any side effects. Keep **ginger biscuits** beside your bed to nibble on when you wake up, or keep **ginger lollipops** in your handbag for those times when you are out and about and your nausea is triggered. You can also chew on **candied ginger** – a 2.5cm piece is equal to about 500–1000mg of **dried ginger**, or take a supplement.

Use **fresh ginger** in smoothies, or add to stir-fries. Another good option to boost your intake is to make **ginger tea** to sip on throughout the day. Steep one teaspoon of grated fresh ginger in boiling water; leave to infuse, then drain and sweeten or dilute more if the taste is too strong. If you prefer not to make your own there are plenty of shop-bought options for ginger tea, too.

Citrus oil morning sickness remedy

As your sense of smell is often heightened in pregnancy, you may find relief from nausea by using essential oils. Morning sickness can strike throughout the day, and this remedy can be used any time you're feeling queasy.

To help settle morning sickness, try using essential oils with a citrus base – **lemon**, **sweet orange**, or **grapefruit**, for example. Less is more when it comes to aromatherapy, so place just one or two drops of your chosen essential oil on a cotton wool ball and take a few deep breaths to inhale the scent. Combine the use of your essential oils and your hypnobirthing practice to create a positive mindset around your pregnancy, and later for your baby's birth – they work wonderfully well together.

"Consult a qualified aromatherapist to find the oil that is most effective for you."

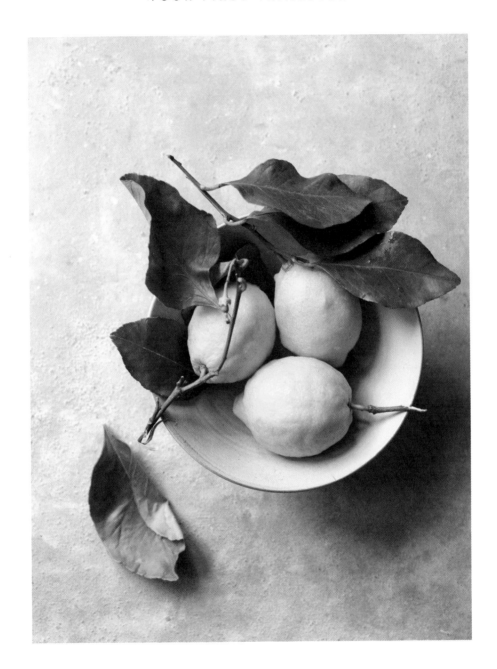

Mini body scan

Throughout pregnancy a constant stream of thoughts can hijack your sense of wellbeing. This simple but powerful exercise calms the brain, relieves anxiety, and is a great way to connect with your growing baby.

1

Sit comfortably on a chair. Bring your attention to the top of your head and slowly begin to move down to your forehead with curiosity.

2

Next, move the spotlight of focus to your cheeks and your jaw. Allow your jaw to open slightly so your tongue rests behind your top teeth.

3

Expand your awareness to your shoulders and allow them to drop down. Notice the middle of your back and the chair supporting you.

4

Bring your attention to your belly where your growing baby is cocooned in serenity, then move your focus down each leg.

5

Extend your awareness to your feet. Notice your connection to the earth and the pull of gravity. Imagine your whole body radiating with a beautiful white light, feeling a deep appreciation for the wisdom and inner intelligence of your amazing body in pregnancy.

"As you pause between each area of your pregnant body, feel gratitude for the incredible work it does every day."

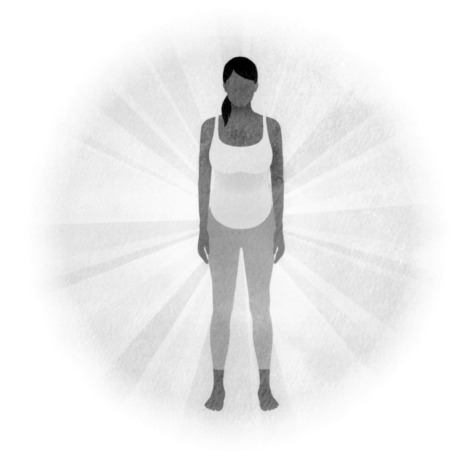

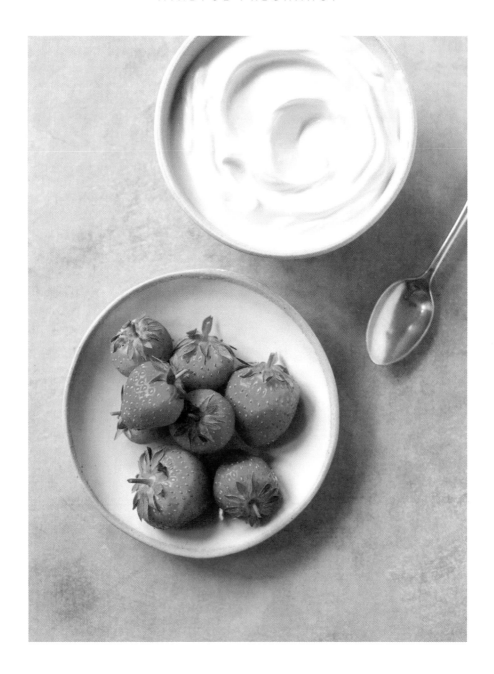

Iodine and choline

Most women consume less than they need of these important nutrients, so you may well need to boost your intake. When shopping and planning meals be mindful about ways you can include more in your diet.

Iodine is important as it makes the thyroid hormones, which are used to regulate all your baby's internal systems including brain development. **Dairy products**, particularly **milk**, and **seafood** such as **cod**, **haddock**, and **plaice** are good sources of iodine, especially if you add **iodized salt** for flavour. For a nutritious snack that's packed with iodine, as well as fibre and minerals, add some **sea lettuce** (Ulva) to a salad once a week, or toast a few leaves with some **sesame seeds**.

Choline is essential for your baby's brain development. Good sources include **lean red meat, fish, chicken, legumes** (beans and peas), **eggs**, and **nuts**. Fresh cod is a tasty dinner option that is rich in choline, and as it's not an oily fish you can eat it more than twice a week. You can also sprinkle **wheatgerm** onto a **yoghurt** or your breakfast cereal or add it to a fruit smoothie to boost your choline levels.

Mindful shower

Enjoying a mindful shower allows you to start or end your day feeling more grounded and present. You can follow these steps at whatever pace your routine allows, connecting with your baby as you focus on your body.

1

As the water is heating up, take a few deep breaths. Step into the shower and engage all of your senses.

2

Notice the sound of the water. Notice the temperature of the water on your skin and appreciate the warmth.

3

Breathe in the scent of your favourite soap or shower gel and appreciate the luxuries in your life.

4

Notice how the warm water washes over your skin, nurturing your changing body and growing baby. Imagine it washing away any tension and stress. If your mind wanders, congratulate yourself for noticing that your attention has moved and relax again into the calming sensations of a warm shower.

5

End your shower with appreciation for your pregnancy and growing baby, and with gratitude for your amazing body.

"*Mindfully showering transforms a routine, everyday task into a replenishing ritual.*"

Vitamin D

Sunlight is the best source of vitamin D, so in the winter you may find yourself deficient in it. However, it is found in a number of foods, including eggs and oily fish, so it's easy to boost your levels by considering your diet.

Vitamin D helps us to absorb the right amount of calcium and phosphate and helps your baby's teeth, bones, kidneys, and heart to develop in the womb. Research also found that women who had good levels of vitamin D were more likely to have an uncomplicated birth, decreasing the chance of having a premature baby or a caesarean birth. You can get vitamin D from a number of foods including **egg yolks**, **oily fish** such as **salmon**, **sardines**, and **herrings**, and **fortified orange juice** and **milk**.

The primary source of vitamin D is sunshine, and vitamin D deficiency is quite common in Northern Europe, particularly in the winter months. If you can get out in the open air for short periods each day you can top up your vitamin D levels without supplementation. A study of UK adults suggests even 13 minutes of sun exposure on the arms and legs, three times a week, supports healthy vitamin D levels. If out in the sun for longer, use a mineral sunscreen to protect you from sun damage while allowing for some vitamin D absorption.

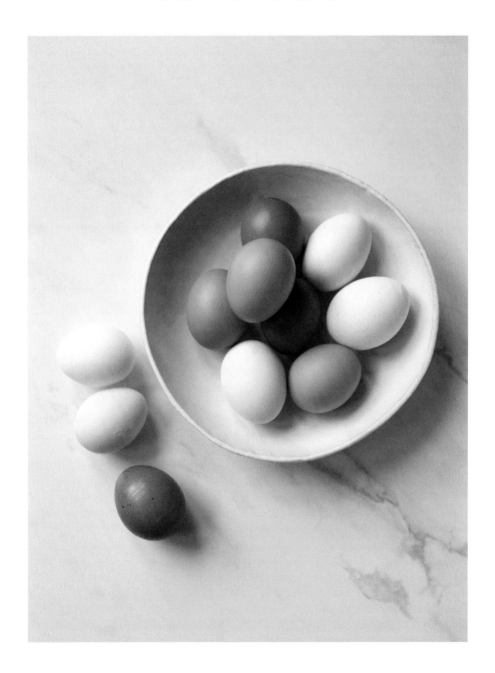

Mindful walking

*Gentle exercise throughout your pregnancy is essential
to your health and your baby's. Daily mindful walks will
allow you to develop more focus while also expanding
your awareness of what's happening in your body.*

1

Stand up and take
a few deep breaths.
Allow yourself to
really experience
what it feels like
to be in your body.

2

Start by walking slowly, so you can really pay
attention to all of the subtle movements involved.
Be aware of the different sensations in your feet:
where your feet connect with the ground, their
temperature, and the sensation of your shoes.
Stay with your feet for a few steps.

3

Connect with your calf muscles as
you lift and replace your feet on the
ground. Take a few steps. Notice how
your knee bends and the way one
foot makes contact with the ground
while the other foot lifts up.

4

As you walk, notice how your
body feels as your hips move. Keep
your focus on the movements in your
pelvis. Feel how one side moves
forward and then the other; one
hip lifts, while the other hip sinks.

5

Notice how your arms swing by your side. Focus next on your belly. Is your baby still or kicking, active or quiet?

6

Notice your rib cage and how it lifts with each breath. Notice how your shoulders move in the opposite way to your hips.

7

Become aware of your neck, the muscles holding your head, and your jaw. Finish by focusing on the top of your head.

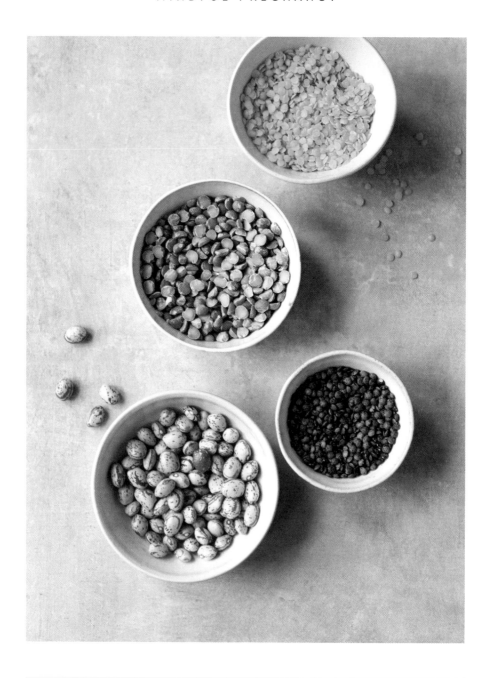

Protein power

Making sure you are eating enough protein every day can help ward off common dietary issues in pregnancy such as carb cravings and unstable blood sugar levels, thus improving your mood and energy levels.

Protein is required for the development of your baby, as well as transporting oxygen and making essential antibodies and hormones. The best sources of protein are **fish**, **meat**, and **poultry**, but **eggs**, **pulses**, and **lentils** are also good sources. If morning sickness is making mealtimes difficult, then a cup of hot **bone broth** is a stomach-friendly, protein-rich drink.

If you want to boost your protein intake, keep a few hard-boiled eggs in the fridge for a quick, healthy snack. Try some **pumpkin seeds**, seasoned **chickpeas,** or **peanut butter** with apple slices or wholegrain crackers for a morning snack. For a delicious lunch or dinner, blend peanut butter with a coconut yoghurt, sweet chilli sauce, and coriander to make a Thai-style dressing for a chicken salad.

Practice and posture

Most yoga experts recommend doing yoga every day, but as a busy and probably tired mum-to-be this may not be realistic in your first trimester. The exercises here can easily be adapted to the time and energy you have.

Tiredness and hormonal surges in the first weeks of pregnancy require a kind approach to your changing body, energy levels, and emotions, so give yourself permission to embrace and accept rest when needed. Some of the yoga positions, such as Hip Circles *(see p72)* and Mountain Pose *(see p69)*, are more energizing than others, while Child's Pose *(see p74)* is an excellent position to help with first trimester fatigue and nausea.

"Antenatal yoga is about mindful connection to your breath, body, and baby – not working up a sweat."

20-MINUTE SEQUENCE

*Start your antenatal yoga practice with this gentle sequence.
Or, if you prefer, do one or two exercises in the morning and
a couple of the more relaxing poses in the evening.*

01

MOUNTAIN POSE

Stand with your feet hip-distance
apart and ground your feet on
your mat. Gently engage your
core abdominal muscles to
stabilize your pelvis. As you
inhale, lengthen through your
torso and elongate your neck.
Your ears, shoulders, hips, and
ankles should all be in one line.
Hold for a few minutes.

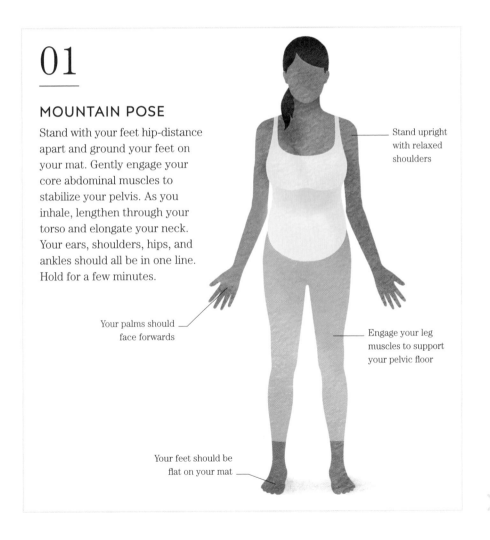

Stand upright
with relaxed
shoulders

Your palms should
face forwards

Engage your leg
muscles to support
your pelvic floor

Your feet should be
flat on your mat

02

EASY POSE

From Mountain Pose, move to a seated position. Sit up straight and tall. Cross your legs comfortably, bringing your feet in towards you. Drop your shoulders, relax your jaw, bring your hands to your belly, and untuck your pelvis. Close your eyes. Inhale peace and exhale worry – use this slow breathing to reduce any anxiety.

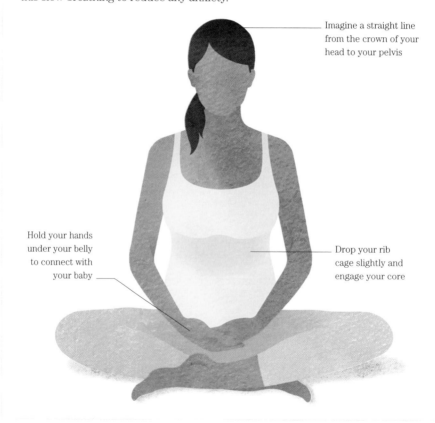

Imagine a straight line from the crown of your head to your pelvis

Hold your hands under your belly to connect with your baby

Drop your rib cage slightly and engage your core

03

TABLETOP

From Easy Pose, move slowly onto your hands and knees. Your knees should be hip-width apart, with your feet directly behind your knees. Align your palms directly under your shoulders with your fingers spread out. Look down between your hands and flatten your back. Press down into your palms. Hold this stabilizing pose for a few minutes.

SUPPORTED WRISTS

Pregnancy hormones can increase carpal tunnel symptoms. If sore, come down onto your forearms.

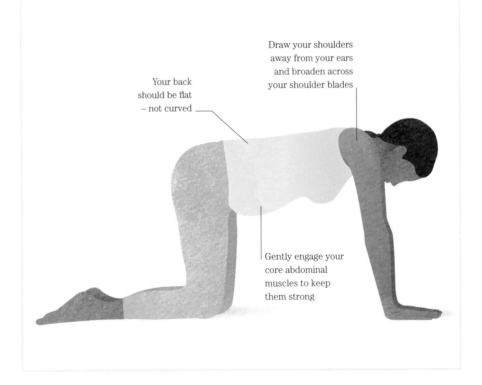

Draw your shoulders away from your ears and broaden across your shoulder blades

Your back should be flat – not curved

Gently engage your core abdominal muscles to keep them strong

04

GOOD FOR
FLEXIBILITY

Hip circles encourage
flexibility in the hips and
lower back and relieve
ligament pain as the
pelvic organs begin
to shift.

HIP CIRCLES

In Tabletop, take several deep breaths and begin gently
and intuitively moving your pelvis back towards your
heels, then around and forwards in big circles. Keep
your elbows soft so you can move more deeply into
the circles, then change the direction or the size of the
circles you are making. This gentle movement will help
to keep your back muscles strong throughout pregnancy.
Continue for a few minutes, then return to Tabletop.

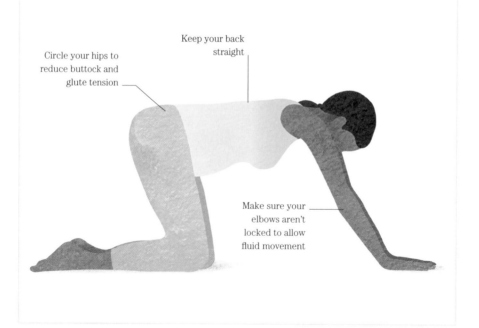

Keep your back
straight

Circle your hips to
reduce buttock and
glute tension

Make sure your
elbows aren't
locked to allow
fluid movement

05

PUPPY POSE

From Tabletop, walk your hands towards the top of your mat, extend your arms fully, and lower your head to the mat to bring a sense of calm. Keep your hands outer-shoulder-width apart. Separate your knees so they are a little wider than your hips. Press your palms down into the floor while keeping your bottom up. Stay in this pose for up to a minute, breathing slowly and deeply into the upper and lower back, and feeling any upper body tension release. Ease out of this relaxing pose slowly and mindfully and return to Tabletop.

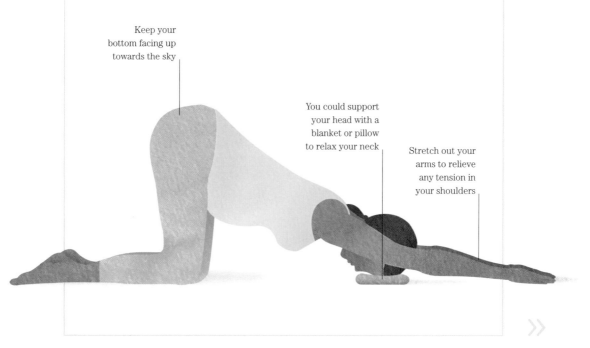

Keep your bottom facing up towards the sky

You could support your head with a blanket or pillow to relax your neck

Stretch out your arms to relieve any tension in your shoulders

06

CHILD'S POSE

From Tabletop, bring your big toes together and spread your knees as wide as is comfortable. Slowly relax your hips down towards your heels and extend your arms towards the front of your mat. Let your forehead rest gently on your mat. You can stretch your arms out in front of you or bend them at the elbow. This is one of the best relaxation positions, so rest for a few minutes and connect to your breath and your baby.

EASES NAUSEA

Child's Pose is a very nurturing position and is excellent for helping with first trimester fatigue and morning sickness.

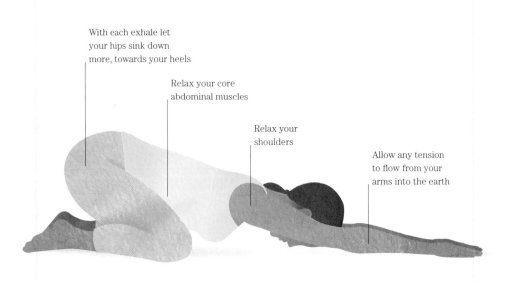

With each exhale let your hips sink down more, towards your heels

Relax your core abdominal muscles

Relax your shoulders

Allow any tension to flow from your arms into the earth

07

RESTING POSE

From Child's Pose, roll slowly onto your side, then over onto your back. Place cushions under your neck and knees for support. Allow your arms and feet to relax outwards, your hands open. Cover yourself with a warm blanket if you wish. Take up to 10 minutes to breathe deeply, following the in breath as it moves through your body, relaxing each muscle. Rest is important in this trimester, so take time to nurture yourself in this pose. When ready, slowly sit up, and then come up to standing.

Focus your attention onto your belly to connect with your baby

Allow the ligaments of your knees and calves to rest comfortably on the supports

Breathe deeply as your body relaxes

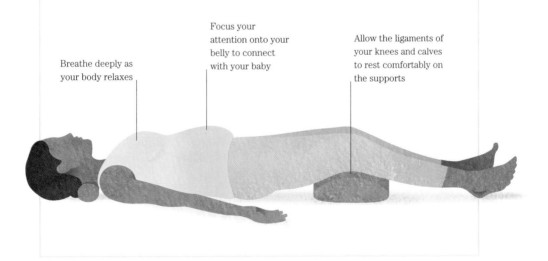

YOUR SECOND TRIMESTER

Weeks 13 to 27 are a very exciting time as your bump grows noticeably and you will feel your baby's first kicks. As your energy returns and any queasiness abates, this is a good time to focus on optimum nutrition, meditation, and mindful movement such as antenatal yoga or mindful walking.

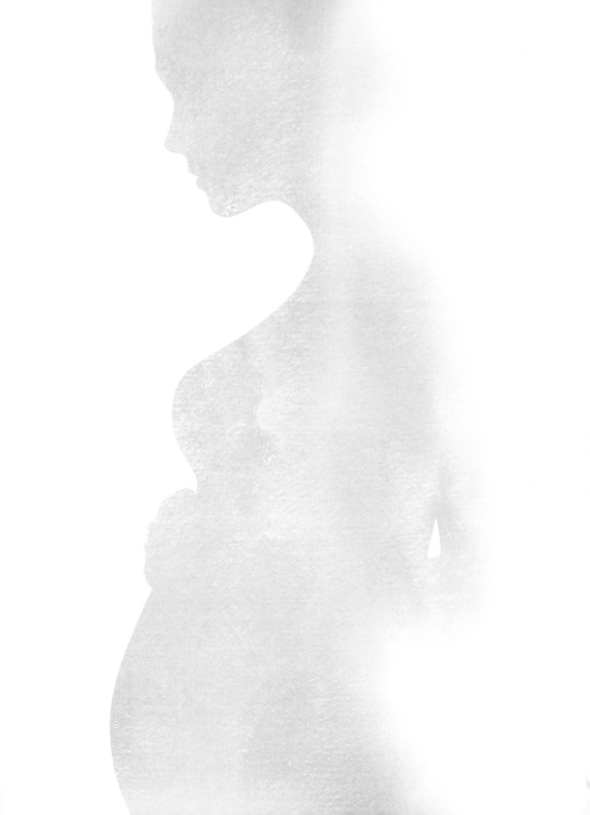

What's happening?

Welcome to your second trimester – a time of glowing and growing! Mindful breathing and short meditations throughout your day will help you feel calmer and more emotionally balanced as your baby's growth accelerates.

Your bump is likely to be showing by now, your hair will probably feel thick and glossy, and it's finally time to tell everyone your good news. With the return of more energy, and hopefully the end of morning sickness, the second trimester is often referred to as the "sweet spot" of pregnancy.

Most mums-to-be are feeling less tired now, so this is a great time to focus on regular, gentle exercise and continuing to eat healthy, nutritious foods *(see p24)*. You may also feel more sexy in this trimester – but don't worry, you won't hurt your baby.

Combining good food and light exercise will help you minimize pregnancy discomforts that are more common during this trimester, such as backache, constipation *(see p94)*, heartburn *(see p84)*, and low iron levels *(see p86)*.

"The most exciting part of this trimester is feeling your baby's first amazing kicks."

All about you

The second trimester is a good time to focus on both hypnobirthing exercises *(see p96)* and meditation techniques *(see p84 and p88)*. These complementary practices have a cumulative effect, so the more that you can practise them throughout your pregnancy, the more you and your baby get to enjoy the benefits of a calmer, more enjoyable pregnancy.

This trimester is also an ideal time to take a holiday as you'll feel most comfortable travelling. The next trip you take will probably be with your baby, so enjoy some rest and relaxation with your partner, taking time to bond and connect, and making plans for your baby's arrival.

All about your baby

In the second trimester your baby's reproductive organs are forming and you may be able to see on a scan if you're expecting a boy or a girl. You might also be able to see your baby sucking his thumb.

Your baby's sense of hearing is beginning to develop, and he can hear your heartbeat, which is reassuring for him before and after birth. If you sing lullabies to your baby throughout your

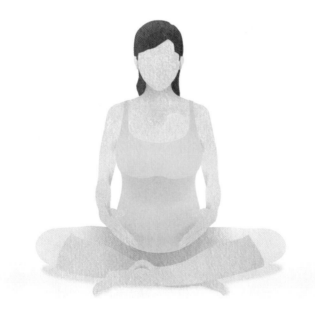

pregnancy he'll recognize the tune and your voice after he's born. Singing to your baby also releases oxytocin, which helps make you both feel good.

Looking ahead

Although it may seem like your baby's due date is far away, this is the perfect time to start considering birth options so don't forget to book your antenatal class and think about hiring a doula. The test when choosing a doula is to ask yourself how you'd feel if you were stuck in a lift with this person for 24 hours. Trust your gut feeling and look for a connection with this important member of your birth team.

Your pelvic floor

It is very normal to worry about your pelvic floor and the sensitive perineum during labour, but there are ways to build strength and flexibility in your pelvic floor, which will support healing after birth. Your pelvic floor muscles act like a "hammock", supporting your bladder, bowel, and uterus. Pregnancy hormones and the growing weight of your baby put a strain on your pelvic floor, and the pushing stage of labour can leave some new mums with temporary pelvic floor changes.

What you need for labour is a flexible, relaxed, supported pelvic floor and that begins with lengthening those muscles. It's common to hear about kegels and pelvic floor "strengthening", but if your buttock muscles (glutes) aren't getting any exercise then that adds to pelvic floor problems. Ideally combine the pelvic floor exercise (*see opposite*) with squatting *(see p107)* every day – the benefits will pay off long after the birth.

"This is the perfect time to cultivate calm with mindful attention to daily activities."

PELVIC FLOOR EXERCISES

Incorporate your pelvic floor exercises into your daily routine, for example, do them whenever you brush your teeth, so you don't have to worry about fitting them in during your day.

1

You can stand or sit to do this exercise. Begin with slow, focused breathing. Concentrate on your pelvic floor muscles (the muscles that you use if you stop your wee mid flow).

2

Imagine that your pelvic floor muscles are a lift. The doors close and the lift goes up to the first floor, then the second floor, and finally the third floor. Tune into your body.

3

Slowly tighten your pelvic floor, lifting the muscles inwards and upwards, remembering to breathe. Continue lifting up, mindfully pausing for five seconds at each "floor".

4

Once you reach the third floor, pause for five seconds, then slowly release the muscles (don't just let go) as you descend floor by floor. It can be hard to hold the squeeze in the beginning, so if necessary build up to five seconds and eventually up to about eight seconds. Slow, focused breathing helps when practising this exercise.

5

Repeat this exercise several times a day, for example, when you put on your makeup, while practising yoga, or even while cooking.

Healthy fats

As you enter the second trimester, your appetite should return. Around 25–35 per cent of your daily calories should come from fats – mindfully choose the right kind of healthy, natural fats and oils for the most benefits.

Fats and oils provide energy and also contain vitamins A, D, E, and K as well as essential fatty acids. Omega-3 fatty acids are especially beneficial for your baby's brain and nervous system. Foods such as **nuts**, **seeds**, **avocados**, and **oils** are good sources of unsaturated fat. **Wild-caught salmon**, **trout**, **sardines**, **mackerel**, and **egg yolks** are particularly high in omega-3 fatty acids; while **soy**, **corn**, and **vegetable oils**, nuts, and seeds are high in omega-6 fatty acids

Boost your omega-3 intake by cooking with **avocado oil** or use it to drizzle over salads. Add a nutty flavour to a lunchtime salad or yoghurt by including **walnuts**. Sardines are an easy way to boost your omega-3 intake (just not more than twice a week). If you don't like fish, then consider taking a **fish oil supplement** to ensure you get enough omega-3.

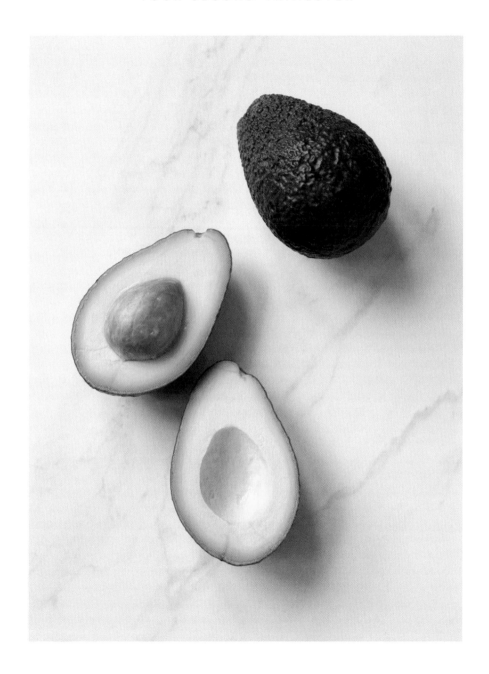

Mindful eating

With your appetite returning in the second trimester, heartburn can be an unwelcome visitor. Eating meals more mindfully and appreciatively may help to reduce heartburn as you slow down and chew your food more.

1

Turn off the TV, phone, etc., and avoid multitasking as you'll miss the cues that you're getting full. Look at your food and breathe in the aroma.

2

Chew slowly and pay attention to the taste, texture, and smell of the food. Notice how your tongue moves the food all around your mouth.

3

Notice the urge to swallow arising, be with that sensation for a moment, then swallow. Take another small bite and mindfully continue.

4

If you find eating slowly is hard to do, put your cutlery down between each bite or put your fork in your non-dominant hand.

5

As you eat, think of all the people involved in bringing this food to your table and mentally thank them. After the exercise notice how different that was to your usual experience of eating: you were fully engaged in the present moment and nothing else mattered but this mindful moment.

"Fully appreciating the food you eat can help you make healthier choices to nourish your baby."

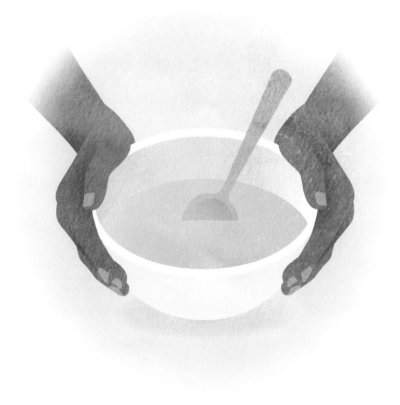

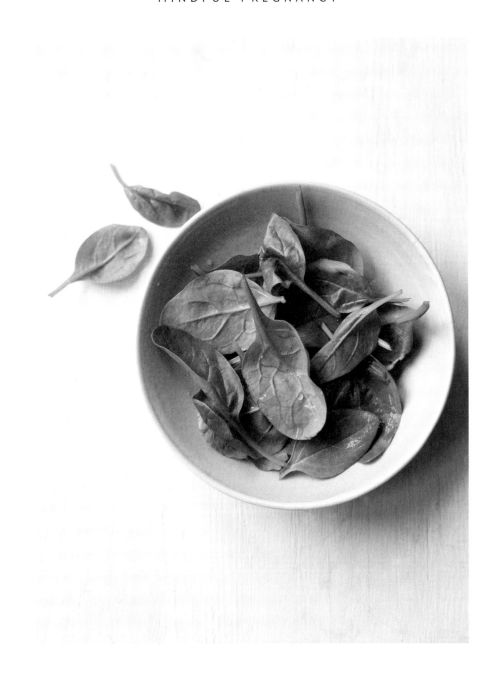

Iron

Crucial for the development of your baby's cells and organs, iron is also needed by the placenta. During pregnancy your blood volume increases, so you (and your baby) need more iron to make red blood cells.

For an iron-rich start to the day, add a couple of **prunes** or some **raisins** to your breakfast cereal and enjoy with a glass of unsweetened orange juice. **Red meat** is a great source of iron, so ideally combine good plant and meat sources – why not have a **steak** with **leafy greens** or **baby spinach**? For non-meat eaters, consider adding even more plant-based iron sources to your diet, such as **dried beans** and **peas**. For an iron-boosting snack, try **pumpkin seeds**, **cashew nuts**, or a **few dried apricots** or **figs**.

If you are lacking iron, combine it with vitamin C to improve absorption – have it with orange juice or include tomatoes in an iron-rich meal. Avoid caffeinated drinks at mealtimes as they inhibit iron absorption. If you decide to take an iron supplement, note it can sometimes cause digestive discomforts, with constipation being the most common side effect *(see also p94)*. If this is the case, talk to your health-care provider.

Cocoon of calm

As you notice those first magical kicks during this trimester, you can deepen the connection with your baby throughout each day. Join your baby whenever you want – in this private space, a refuge of serenity.

1

Sit or lie comfortably and simply focus on your breath. Breathe in confidence and breathe out stress. Breathe in love and breathe out worry.

2

Imagine that a beautiful light is just over your head. This radiant light of wellbeing moves down over your head, relaxing your forehead, before moving towards your shoulders. It is surrounding you in a blanket of tranquility and protection. It envelops you completely, swirling around you gently – a luminous cocoon of peace and calm.

3

Inside this cocoon all is quiet and calm; like the eye of the storm. You can step into this cocoon whenever you need to. Leave any noise and distractions behind you. This is your sanctuary – all that is here is your soft breathing and your baby.

4

If you drift away from focusing on your breath, gently guide your attention back to your breathing.

5

Focus on experiencing this deep calmness. You can take this sanctuary of inner calm and confidence with you as you move through your day. Any time you need to drop into this sanctuary, just repeat to yourself: "Cocoon of calm ... cocoon of calm" and take a few slow, deep breaths as you are enveloped in that radiant light of peace and compassionate awareness.

Coconut oil for massage

Daily massage with coconut oil will nourish the skin, may help to reduce stretch marks, and will ease any itchiness. Start this mindful practice in your second trimester and continue it throughout your pregnancy.

Massage is a calming, nurturing way to connect with your body in pregnancy and promotes the release of oxytocin, a powerful feel-good hormone that you and your baby both experience during a massage. As your bump begins to bloom, gentle abdominal massage is a simple way to bond with your baby – indeed, many mums report feeling their baby kick when they massage their bumps in the later trimesters. This is a nurturing practice you and your partner can do together. Play some music and talk to your baby during the massage – she will learn to recognize your voices.

For the massage, sit between your partner's legs or sit upright on your bed with lots of pillows for support. Apply **coconut oil** or **sweet almond oil** to your hands, then using the flats of your hands, slowly move up from your pubic bone and around your bump gently massaging in circles with slow, focused breathing.

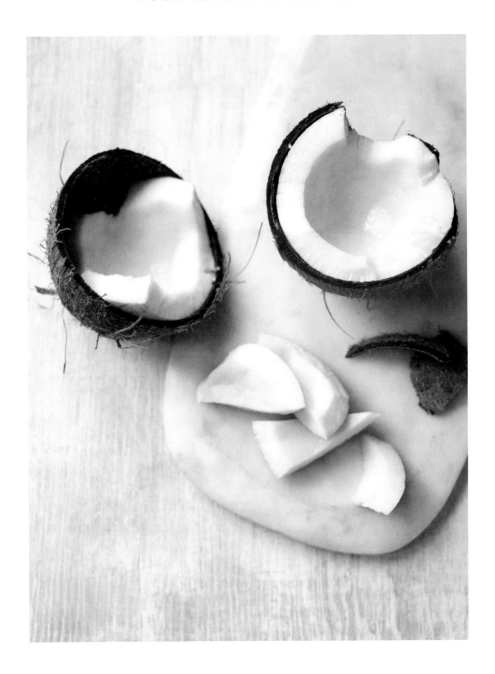

Humming bee breath

As your body continues to change, practise this simple breathing technique every day to keep your mind calm and clear. It brings rich oxygenated blood to your baby as well as making a reassuring vibration.

1

Sit in a comfortable position. Take a few deep, cleansing breaths or make a few loud sighs while you settle yourself.

2

When ready, on the next nourishing breath inhale deeply, and then as you exhale through your nose make the buzzing sound of a bee, low and continuous. You will feel the vibration throughout your body, as will your baby in the womb.

3

Inhale and exhale, making the nasal buzzing sound on each exhale.

4

Continue for a few breaths, until you feel completely relaxed, calm, and settled. If you use this technique now, your baby will become familiar with it, and it can be used to settle him after birth, by making the buzzing sound as you cuddle him.

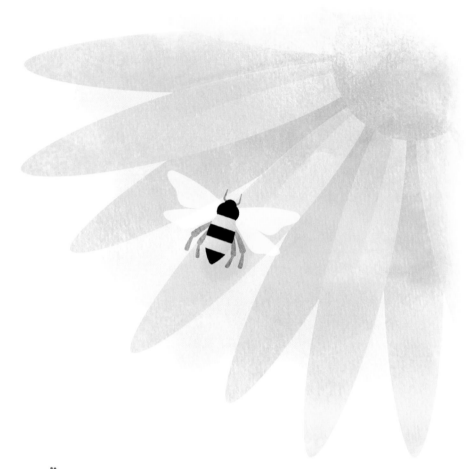

"If you're feeling overwhelmed, close your eyes and block your ears so you can focus only on the buzzing sound."

Fibre

The action of your gut slows down when you are pregnant. It's important you eat enough fibre to prevent it from slowing down too much, causing constipation, a common digestive challenge this trimester.

You can minimize the risk of becoming constipated with some simple dietary changes as well as regular exercise and adequate hydration. Start by adding **bran**, **nuts**, **wholegrain breads**, **crackers**, and low-sugar wholegrain breakfast **cereals** to your diet. Slowly increase the amount of fibre, though, so your body adapts gently. **Fruits** and **berries** are great options, too. **Figs** and **pears** are high in fibre and other essential nutrients and are often overlooked. Start your day with a fibre-packed breakfast of **oatmeal** with added pear slices and **raspberries**, which will also help to keep your blood sugar in check.

Feeling peckish? Try freeze-dried **edamame**, a small packet of unsweetened **trail mix**, or some guilt-free air-popped **popcorn** and a couple of pieces of **dark chocolate**. You'll enjoy these "treats" even more if you savour each bite. It can be tempting to use a laxative if suffering from constipation, but check with your health-care provider before you do so.

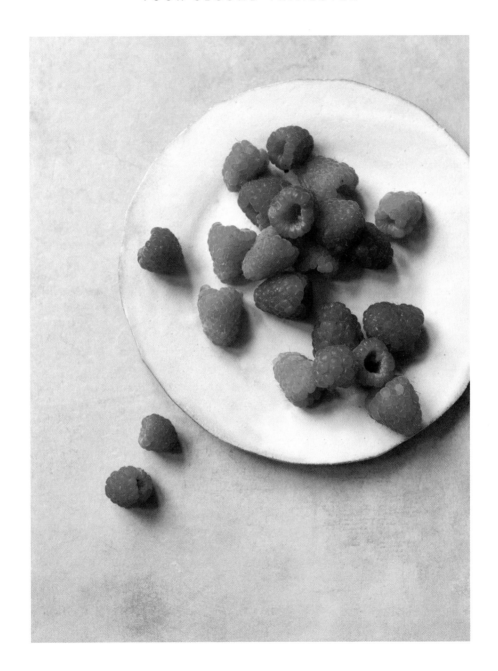

Positive affirmations

As your bump grows, you may be feeling a wide range of emotions. Positive affirmations help keep your mindset uplifted and focused. Choose affirmations that resonate with you (see opposite for ideas) and repeat them daily.

Today, I choose
joy. I give and
receive joy
generously.

I mindfully
choose healthy,
nutritious
foods.

I am strong
in both mind
and body.

I make the right
choices for my
baby and me by
trusting my
inner wisdom.

I feel great
when I exercise
regularly and
take care
of myself.

I am prepared
for whatever
path our
journey
takes us on.

I love and
accept my
changing body.

I speak kindly
to myself.

My baby and
I deserve a
gentle birth.

Essential oils for insomnia

Disrupted sleep is very common during pregnancy, so work out which essential oils are best for you, and use them as part of your bedtime wind-down to ensure you have a good night's sleep.

Finding the right essential oil is crucial as some have a stimulating effect, making it even harder to sleep. The most popular and safest oils for pregnancy that have a relaxing effect include **German** and **Roman chamomile**, **lavender** (but be careful if you have low blood pressure), and **ylang-ylang**.

Adopt a bedtime routine that helps your mind and body to settle down, such as a warm bath with a few drops of essential oil in it; and/or a gentle foot rub or back massage, perhaps from your partner, using essential oils in the massage lotion. You can also put a drop of lavender on a tissue next to your pillow to help you to sleep. Talk to a qualified aromatherapist to find the most effective and safest insomnia blend for you.

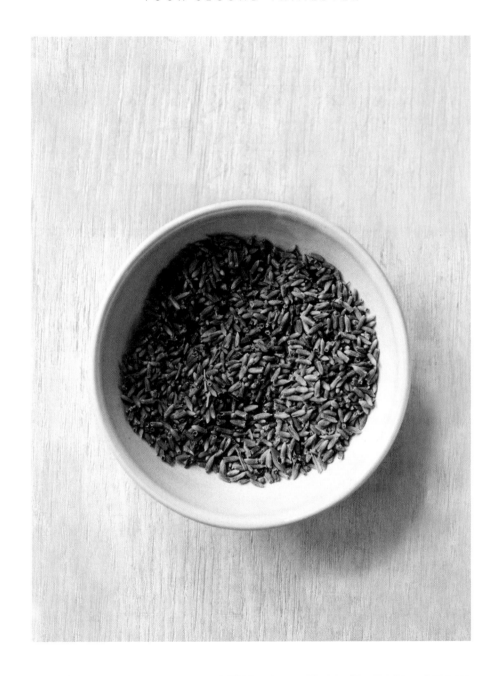

Practice and posture

As you are likely to have more energy in the second trimester, this is the perfect time to extend your yoga sequence. Your body will change rapidly though, so a pose that feels easy early on may become trickier later.

This trimester is the ideal time to cultivate awareness of the present moment with mindful movement through yoga. As physical changes accelerate, focus on slowing your yoga movements for stability and balance. Although you may feel like you can increase your activity levels this trimester, the hormone relaxin adds to your body's flexibility in pregnancy, so make sure you support your joints with the use of blocks, cushions, or blankets so you can modify the poses to your comfort level. Working with your breath is also important as you practise becoming more grounded and centred.

"Approach this trimester with an attitude of appreciation for the intelligence of your body."

30-MINUTE SEQUENCE

A mindful pregnancy and motherhood means weaving these yoga practices into your busy daily life. If time is tight or energy low, break down the sequence so you practise some of the standing, seated, or all-fours poses throughout the day.

01

MOUNTAIN POSE

Stand with your feet hip-distance apart and your arms by your sides, palms facing forwards. Ground your feet, ensuring you are well-balanced as your centre of balance will change as your bump grows. As you inhale, lengthen through your torso and elongate your neck. Hold for a few minutes.

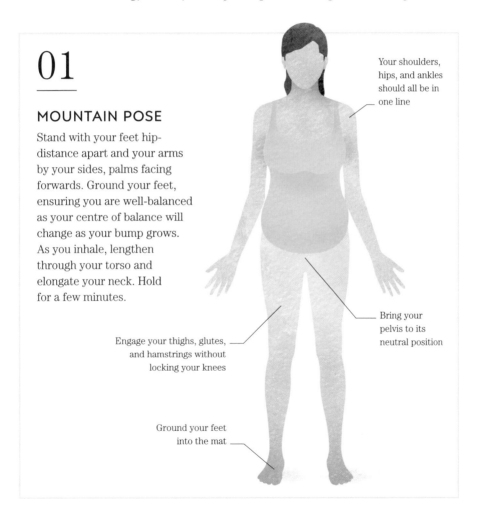

Your shoulders, hips, and ankles should all be in one line

Bring your pelvis to its neutral position

Engage your thighs, glutes, and hamstrings without locking your knees

Ground your feet into the mat

〉〉

02

STANDING TURN I

Begin in Mountain Pose, making sure your feet are hip-width apart. Stretch your arms out to make a T shape. Take a deep breath and, as you exhale, gently turn your upper body to the right. Follow with your head but do not twist your neck to look behind you. Repeat slowly on each side for several deep breaths. Focus on slowing your yoga movements this trimester for stability and balance as your bump grows.

ENERGIZING TURNS

These gentle standing turns reduce the risk of constipation in pregnancy by stimulating your digestive system.

Turn from your rib cage to create space – never twist the abdomen

Keep your hips square

Push your feet into the ground

03

STANDING TURN II

Turn to one side and raise your front arm towards the ceiling, allowing a gentle stretch of the arms and rib cage. As you turn, lift your heel off the mat. Drop your back arm down with the palm of your hand facing down. Take a deep breath in. As you exhale, turn slowly back towards the starting position and bring your arms down to your sides. Repeat for several breaths on each side.

Activate your arm muscles as you slowly turn

Open up your chest to allow for deeper breathing

Stretch your leg muscles by lifting your heel off the mat

04

STANDING TURN III

Begin in Mountain Pose, then bring your palms together in front of your heart. Take a few breaths and imagine a light filling your heart as you breathe in. Inhale as you gently turn from your rib cage to one side, then slowly turn back to the front on the exhale. Repeat on the opposite side.

Do not turn from your abdomen – focus on twisting from your upper back and rib cage

Your palms should be pressed together with your fingers facing up

Keep your knees relaxed so there is flexion in the soft tissues of the knees

05

STANDING TURN IV

As you inhale, gently raise your arms over your head to stretch your upper body and back, while opening the chest. Gently turn to one side. Exhale slowly as you return to Mountain Pose, allowing your arms to float down to your sides. Repeat on the other side for several breaths. Roll your shoulders back a few times to finish.

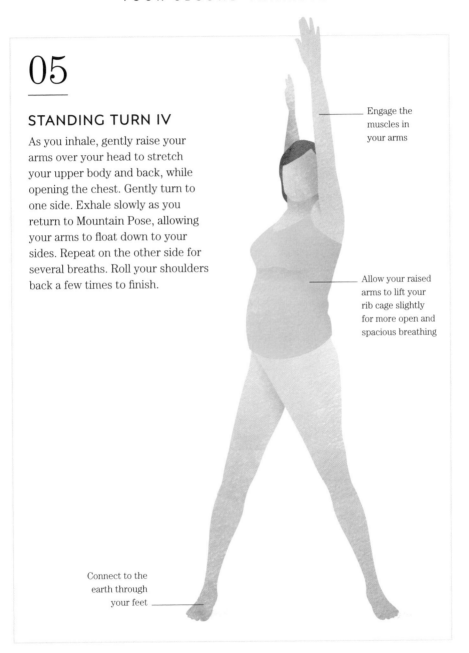

Engage the muscles in your arms

Allow your raised arms to lift your rib cage slightly for more open and spacious breathing

Connect to the earth through your feet

06

WARRIOR POSE

From Mountain Pose, exhale as you step your feet wide apart. Turn your left foot out 90 degrees. Turn your upper body to follow the direction of your toes. Inhale and lift your arms up. Exhale and bend your left knee. Turn your head to follow your body and hold for 20 seconds. Inhale, straighten your knee, and return to Mountain Pose. Pause, then repeat on the other side.

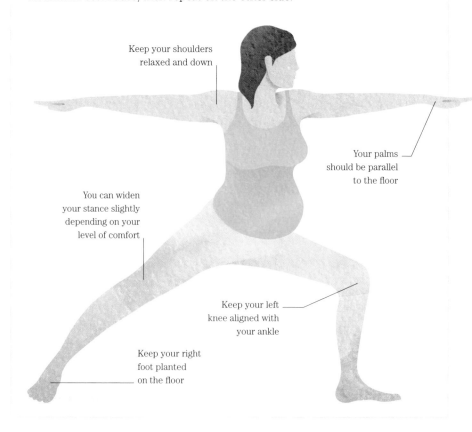

Keep your shoulders relaxed and down

Your palms should be parallel to the floor

You can widen your stance slightly depending on your level of comfort

Keep your left knee aligned with your ankle

Keep your right foot planted on the floor

07

SQUAT

From Mountain Pose, move your feet so they are about shoulder-width apart. Place a folded blanket under your heels and two blocks behind you. Angle your toes towards the corners of your mat and bring your hands to your heart. Inhale as you slowly lower your hips onto the blocks, then exhale as you stand. Engage your pelvic floor. Repeat three times. This pose maintains strength and flexibility in the pelvic floor muscles, hips, glutes, and core as you begin to carry more weight in your pelvis.

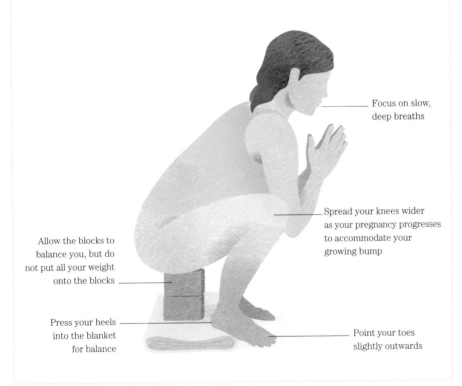

Focus on slow, deep breaths

Spread your knees wider as your pregnancy progresses to accommodate your growing bump

Allow the blocks to balance you, but do not put all your weight onto the blocks

Press your heels into the blanket for balance

Point your toes slightly outwards

08 TABLETOP

Slowly move to your hands and knees: knees apart, hands aligned under your shoulders. Engage your core so your back is flat. Hold for several breaths.

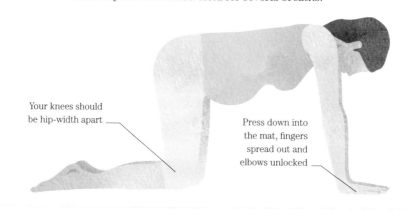

Your knees should be hip-width apart

Press down into the mat, fingers spread out and elbows unlocked

09 HIP CIRCLES

Gently move your pelvis back towards your calves and then forwards in a clockwise motion for at least two breaths, then move in an anticlockwise direction.

Your head and neck should be aligned with your spine

Begin with small hip circles, then widen for a more satisfying stretch

Keep your elbows soft and unlocked

10 CAT

From Tabletop, slowly exhale and lift your ribs. Arch your back like a cat, bringing your chin towards your chest. Return to Tabletop. Repeat several times.

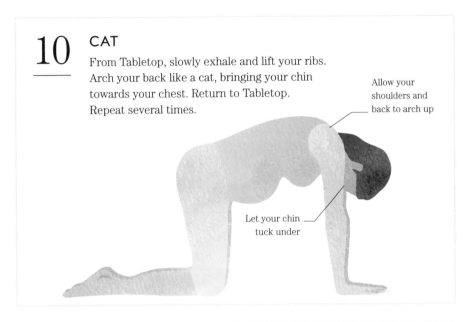

Allow your shoulders and back to arch up

Let your chin tuck under

11 COW

From Tabletop, draw your belly button up towards your spine, keeping your spine aligned with your neck. This helps strengthen your back muscles.

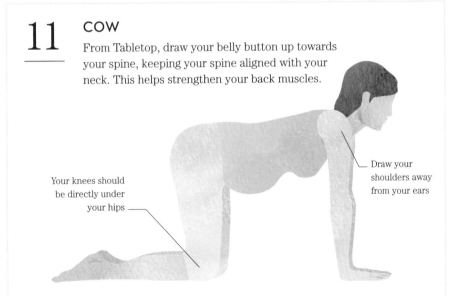

Draw your shoulders away from your ears

Your knees should be directly under your hips

12

ADAPTATION

If you find this pose challenging with your bump, hold onto a secure chair with your hands, instead of bending right down to the floor.

DOWNWARD DOG

This is a great stretching and strengthening pose to energize you this trimester. From Tabletop, press down into your hands. Tilt your tailbone up and tuck your toes under. Lift your hips up, bringing your chest back towards your thighs. Let the weight come from the front of your body back into the hips. Stay in the pose for several breaths. To finish, exhale, drop your knees slowly to the mat as your shoulders move back, and return to Tabletop.

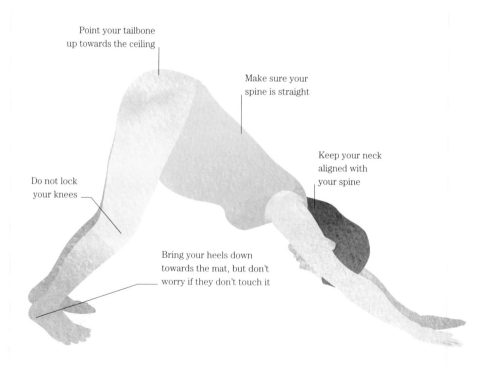

Point your tailbone up towards the ceiling

Make sure your spine is straight

Keep your neck aligned with your spine

Do not lock your knees

Bring your heels down towards the mat, but don't worry if they don't touch it

13

PUPPY POSE

From Tabletop, walk your hands towards the top of your mat, extend your arms fully, and lower your head to the mat. Open your knees wide enough to make space for your growing bump. Press your palms down into the mat, keeping your bottom up. You can use a bolster or pillow to support your forehead. If your wrists are sore, place your forearms on blocks. Hold this calming, nurturing pose for up to a minute, then come back to Tabletop slowly and mindfully by walking your hands back towards you.

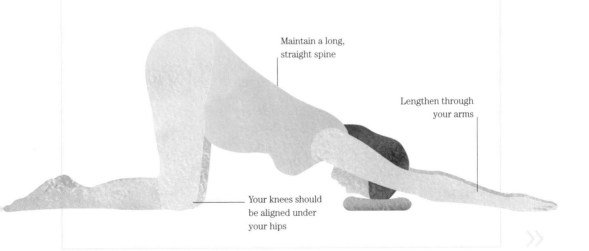

Maintain a long, straight spine

Lengthen through your arms

Your knees should be aligned under your hips

111

14

PIGEON POSE I

From Tabletop, place a bolster in front of you and slowly slide your left knee forwards between your hands and rest on your left hip. Using your hand to help position you, bring your left foot towards your right hip and then square both hips to the ground and straighten your right leg behind you. If you wish, add a blanket or pillow under your left thigh to keep your hips open and place your fingers on the bolster for balance, leaning forwards slightly. Stay here for several breaths, then repeat on the other side.

PAIN RELIEF

Pigeon Pose helps to open up the hips, relieving the common pregnancy problems of sciatica and tension in the lower back and buttocks.

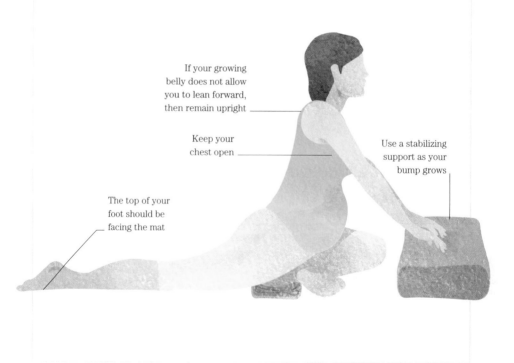

If your growing belly does not allow you to lean forward, then remain upright

Keep your chest open

Use a stabilizing support as your bump grows

The top of your foot should be facing the mat

15

PIGEON POSE II

Try a deeper stretch, allowing an even better expansion of the pelvis, hips, and lower back muscles. From Pigeon Pose I, try to bring your left foot towards your belly. Come down onto your forearms onto the mat, or use a bolster to raise the floor up to you. Breathe in and out for several breaths, allowing your hips to sink down, then return to Tabletop. Repeat on the other side.

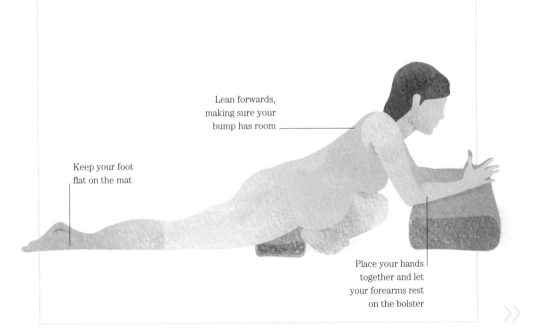

Lean forwards, making sure your bump has room

Keep your foot flat on the mat

Place your hands together and let your forearms rest on the bolster

16

CHILD'S POSE

From Tabletop, bring your big toes together and spread your knees as wide as is comfortable. Relax your hips down towards your heels and extend your arms towards the front of your mat, placing a bolster under your chest and head. Bend your arms at the elbow and hug the bolster. Close your eyes, rest for a few minutes, and connect to your baby. This pose is also an ideal way to relax before you go to bed, combining meditation, breathing, and stretching.

CALMING

Emotional highs and lows are common throughout pregnancy, so use this calming pose to nurture, ground, and relax you.

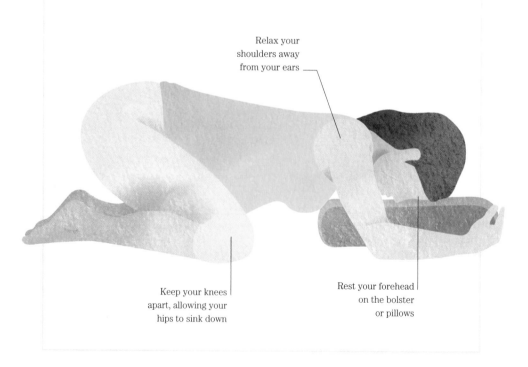

Relax your shoulders away from your ears

Keep your knees apart, allowing your hips to sink down

Rest your forehead on the bolster or pillows

17

SIDE-LYING RESTING POSE

From Child's Pose, roll slowly onto your left-hand side and straighten out your legs. Place a pillow under your head and another pillow or blankets between your legs, then shift your top leg forwards. Tuck a rolled blanket behind your back and under your bump if needed. Close your eyes and focus on your breathing or a visualization. Stay here for about 10 minutes, connecting with your baby, then come out of this pose slowly to avoid dizziness – sitting up first, then standing.

Place a pillow or folded blankets between your slightly bent knees

Place your arm on top of your leg or cradle your bump

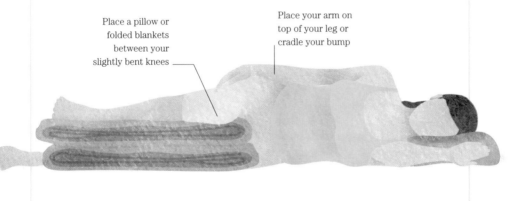

"This relaxing pose calms your nervous system as you rest."

YOUR
THIRD
TRIMESTER

The last weeks of pregnancy can feel emotionally and physically intense as your body gets ready for your baby's arrival. As these changes demand a slower, more purposeful approach to life, you also have a wonderful opportunity to connect with your inner wisdom as you prepare for a positive, mindful birth.

What's happening?

Cultivating calm through mindful practices will help you embrace the huge changes of this trimester, and prepare you mentally for becoming a mother, as well as alleviating any concerns you may have about the birth.

As your pregnancy progresses it's natural for your focus to move to the big day. This can be a physically and mentally demanding time with the business of preparing for your baby's arrival, but keep up your gentle exercise and stay tuned into messages from your body. Really indulge yourself during the third trimester. Take lots of naps, practise the hypnobirthing exercises (*see p132, p134, and p140*), meditate (*see p122, p128, and p138*), and read a great book or two. Make self-care and rest a priority, especially as restorative sleep can be hard to come by now.

If you haven't experienced the bliss of pregnancy massage now is the time to. A gentle, nurturing massage relieves tired muscles and increases levels of the feel-good hormone oxytocin. It's also time for another form of massage

"This is a time for guiltless self-care — it's good for you and for your baby."

– perineal massage *(see p130)*. If you're a first-time mum you can increase your chances of keeping a healthy and (maybe intact) perineum by getting used to the sensation of perineal stretching before labour.

Mindful breathing will be your best friend in labour, so get in lots of practice by using breathing techniques to minimize any aches and pains over the coming weeks *(see p126)*.

If you'd like to have a keepsake of your pregnancy to honour the awe-inspiring work your body is doing, then a belly cast is a great idea, or have professional maternity photos taken.

All about your baby

Your baby is in the final stages of preparation for life outside of the womb. Growth slows in the last few weeks, although it might not feel like it to you. Your baby also lays down brown fat stores which her body uses for heat in the early days if she gets cold (that's why newborns don't shiver).

Your baby is "practising" breathing movements and she may even be dreaming during her short sleep cycles. Her hair is beginning to grow as are her eyebrows and eyelashes. Vernix, a waxy white coating, covers your baby's skin. This "baby butter" has protective

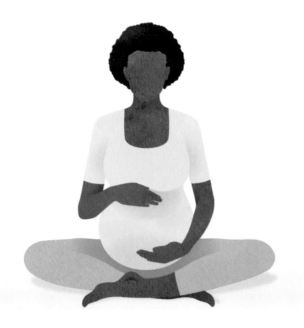

properties for your baby so there is no need to wash it off. Most babies also turn into the head down (vertex) position in the last few weeks in preparation for the journey ahead.

Preparing for a mindful birth

One of the most important factors in how you experience labour, and how your baby arrives, is influenced by who you choose as your primary care provider and where you choose to give birth. A mindful birth can happen in hospital, at home, or a birth centre – all are safe options for healthy mums.

As you continue to cultivate a mindful approach to your baby's birth, consider all the options so that you feel your chosen care provider and place of birth has the skills, resources, and facilities to support a mindful birth. For healthy mums and babies, midwives are the recommended lead care provider for antenatal care, labour, and the postpartum period. It's important to find a care provider who shares your mindful approach to pregnancy and birth, so keep looking until you find the right one.

A knowledgeable, loving birth partner is essential for a mindful birth. When choosing a birth partner (or partners) pay attention to the kind of energy they bring – will they be a calm, nurturing presence or an anxious one? They should facilitate the optimal environment and be a rock for you.

Make sure you and your birth partner take a comprehensive class so you feel ready to welcome your baby together, calmly and confidently. Also read the chapter on labour (*see pp158–189*) so you can feel prepared, with mindful practices in place.

"What your brain is doing in labour is just as important as what your body and baby are doing."

PLANNING AHEAD

Being organized in the lead-up to the birth will make the first few weeks easier. Newborns don't need much, but feeling prepared will help to soothe any last-minute nerves.

Prepare for the birth

Read up about labour (*see pp158–189*) so you feel ready for the birth, and test out your baby equipment. Pack a hospital bag (even if you're planning a home birth) and don't forget to include any hypnobirthing recordings, essential oils (*see p168*), and homeopathic remedies (*see p174*).

"Ready meals"

Stock up your freezer with healthy meals that will encourage healing, good milk supply, and energy after the birth (*see p198*).

Nights out

Have date nights with your partner. Arrange to see your friends as it may be a while before you feel like socializing again.

Be prepared for feeding

Go to a breastfeeding class and support group so you feel more confident about feeding when your baby arrives.

Read up about sleep

Learn about newborn behaviour, especially sleep patterns (*see p192*), so you have realistic expectations.

Communicate

Finalize your birth preferences and chat to your midwife and your partner about how you'd like to be supported during labour.

Get organized

Talk to your partner about a post-birth plan. Split up the household chores – noting that your list should be almost empty!

Doula?

If you won't have a partner to support you, consider hiring a postpartum doula, who will take care of you as a new mother.

Full body scan

As the end of your pregnancy journey approaches, take time to deepen the connection with your body and baby further. Enjoy this appreciative body scan as you prepare to sleep, and notice how your mind settles.

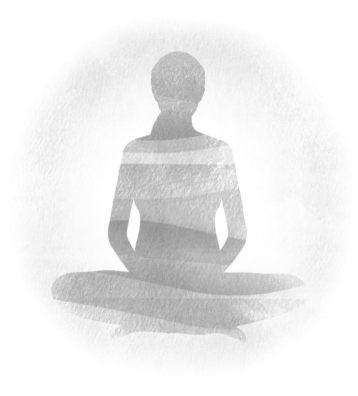

1

Sit or lie comfortably and close your eyes. Focus on any sensations in the toes of your right foot. Imagine each breath flowing into your toes.

2

Move your focus to the sole of your right foot and imagine each breath flowing all the way down to your foot, then repeat with your right ankle. As thoughts come up, let them drift away like a cloud in the sky. There is no need to follow those thoughts, simply bring your awareness back to that place of stillness where you can access so much wisdom.

3

Move your focus to your calf, knee, thigh, and then hip. Repeat the same sequence for your left leg. Move up through your lower back and abdomen, and spend some time noticing your baby's movements, connecting silently with your baby. Notice your upper back, chest, and shoulders, paying attention to the areas of your body that may be uncomfortable. Then focus on the parts that are soft and comfortable.

4

Move your focus to the fingers on your right hand, then move up to your wrist, forearm, elbow, and shoulder. Repeat for your left arm, then move your attention over your neck and throat, and onto your jaw.

5

When you reach the top of your head, imagine your breath moving out beyond your body, cocooning you in calmness. Take a moment of gratitude to appreciate all the work your body does, then open your eyes slowly.

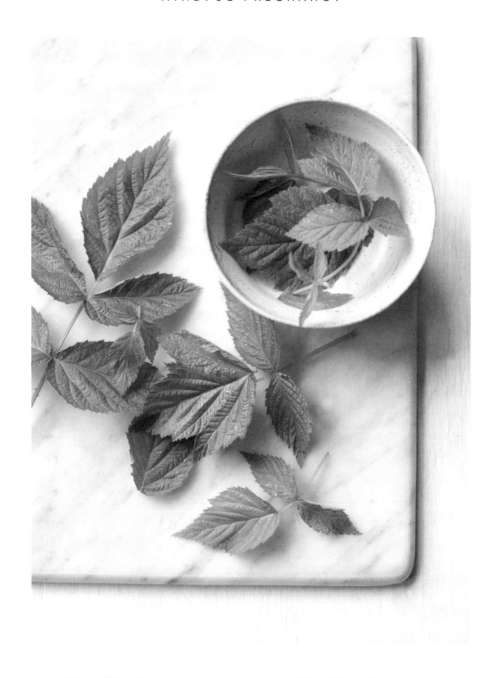

Raspberry leaf tea

This herbal tea is a staple for many expectant mums, and should be introduced slowly only from the third trimester. It won't actually induce labour, but it may reduce your need for intervention in labour.

Raspberry leaf tea is thought to tone the muscles of the uterus and shorten the pushing stage during labour. Start with just one cup a day from the third trimester, and see how your digestive system reacts. Increase to two to three cups as you get closer to your due date. It is also available in capsule form. However, there is some debate on which method confers the most benefits.

When the weather is hot, why not try **iced raspberry leaf tea**? Pour boiling water over four or five tea bags and steep for five minutes (or longer if you like a stronger flavour). Pour the tea into a glass jug and allow to cool. Add one cup of cold water to the jug and store in the fridge. Either drink it as it is, experiment adding fruit such as lemon or orange wedges, or add manuka honey if you prefer it sweeter.

Relaxing breath

The third trimester is the perfect time to start focusing on slow, intentional breathing, so practise this exercise every day if possible. It will help you to feel more emotionally stable and will be invaluable during labour.

1

Either stand or sit. Start with the word "relax", and notice how it is made up of two syllables: "re" and "lax".

2

As you breathe in, think "re", and as you breathe out, think "lax". Try to lengthen your out breath so the second part is longer: "re-laaaaaaaaax".

3

Keep your attention focused solely on that one word, slowly repeating the word "relax" in tune with your breathing.

4

Focus again on lengthening the out breath; the in breath will take care of itself.

5

Imagine seeing those letters written in the sand on a warm, white sandy beach. As you breathe in you see the gentle waves approaching and washing over those letters. As you breathe out that "wave" of breath washes away any worries you may have. Practise often as you prepare for a mindful birth.

"For best effects, combine breathing techniques with relaxing imagery."

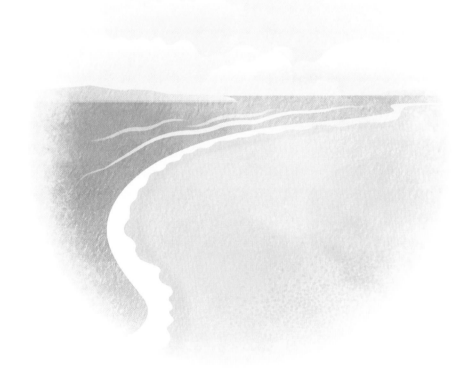

Compassion meditation

The third trimester can bring up challenging feelings. Doing a simple, loving-kindness meditation every day means that you can meet these emotions with an open heart and feel more connected to those around you.

1

Sit upright and soften your gaze or close your eyes. Focus on your breathing. Notice the pause between breaths; between the inhale and the exhale.

2

Spend a few moments retrieving the image of someone who really loves you: your partner, best friend, a grandparent, or even a family pet. Imagine they are sitting next to you and allow yourself to deeply feel their love, kindness, and compassion for you. Bask in those feelings.

3

As you feel those wonderful emotions imagine sending yourself positive, loving thoughts. Say to yourself silently the following intentions: "May I be healthy and well. May I be happy. May I be filled with ease."

4

Next, think of someone you feel neutral towards. Imagine sending them those same positive intentions.

5

Now bring to mind someone you do not feel positive towards. Bring your focus back to your breathing and repeat the same positive intentions.

6

Finally send the same intentions out to the world, widening your circle of compassion to all beings. Silently repeat: "May all beings everywhere be healthy and well. May all beings be happy. May all beings be filled with ease."

Almond oil for perineal massage

Regular perineal massage from about 36 weeks to birth reduces the risk of perineal tearing in labour. Do this for 10 minutes a few times a week using almond oil, which is moisturizing and packed with vitamin E.

Perineal massage gently stretches the skin and tissues around the opening of the vagina and perineum and helps you get used to the sensation of stretching in the perineal tissues. In an unmedicated birth that sensation provides feedback to you to breathe slowly and relax into the brief but powerful sensations, rather than tensing up and pushing harder. The slower and more controlled the emergence of your baby's head, the less likely you'll experience perineal injury.

Rub **almond oil** or any **unscented organic oil** onto your fingers, thumbs, and the outside of your perineum. Place your thumbs 5mm inside your vagina. Press down (toward the anus) and to the sides until you feel a slight burning sensation. Hold for one minute. With your thumbs, slowly massage the lower half of the vaginal opening using a "U" shaped movement.

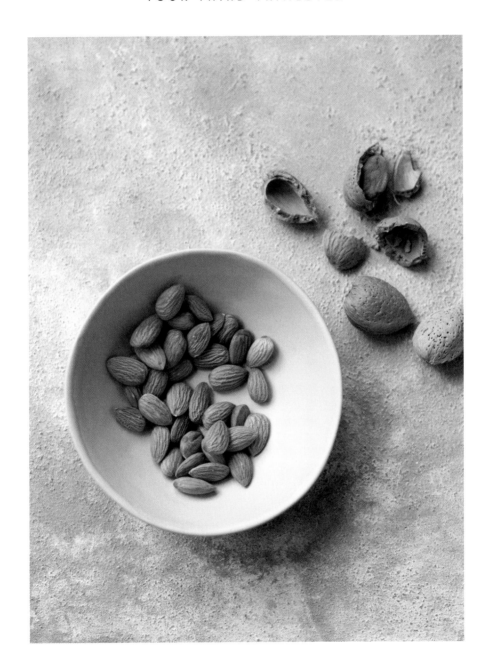

Birth visualization

If this visualization speaks to you, soothe any nerves by reading through it at least once a day, adapting the imagery to your unique birth vision. Allow the scenes to play out as you get excited about meeting your baby.

1

Lie down and take a few deep breaths. Notice the sensations within your body. Everything is calm, relaxed, and safe.

2

Starting with your toes, allow a wave of relaxation to move up over your entire body as if you're being covered by a blanket. Imagine you're taking a walk on a quiet, secluded beach. You can hear the waves and smell the salty sea air, bringing back childhood memories. Let your imagination engage your senses.

3

See the gentle waves washing up onto the sand and receding back towards the ocean. Enjoy the hypnotic rhythm. And just like the waves, your surges will come and go rhythmically: building, swelling, peaking, and then dissipating. Between these waves, relax completely and re-energize.

4

You are excited that these surging waves of energy are bringing your baby to you, each rolling wave, one after the other.

5

Allow the waves
to carry you and
your baby safely – your
baby sliding through
the soft tissues with
each wave. And at any
point you and your
baby can float down
effortlessly and
dreamily into an
underwater world.

6

Imagine your baby
in the perfect position
for a gentle birth.
Your body and baby
are working in
harmony for a calm,
confident delivery. As
your baby's head
slowly emerges almost
unnoticed, you relax
fully and completely.

7

Imagine those first
moments holding your
baby. Feel the weight
of your baby in your
arms, skin-to-skin.
Imagine the moment
your eyes first lock –
a moment of joy,
recognition, and love
as you meet each
other on the outside.

Magical forest

Practise this exercise daily during the third trimester if you find this visualization resonates with you (or see p132 for an alternative), so you can connect with your baby in the coming weeks and during the birth process.

1

Count slowly from 10 down to one. Imagine you are in a beautiful forest. The deeper into the forest you go, the more you relax.

2

You feel at one with the forest and nature. As you absorb the stillness and beauty, you can feel any tension draining away.

3

A clearing appears, and wrapped in a blanket is your baby, coming to meet you from the future, her arms outstretched.

4

Go to your baby and pick her up. Breathe in her deliciousness. Explore her tiny fingers and toes. Touch her downy hair.

5

Your baby's eyes meet yours and you're overcome by the feeling that you have known each other for a lifetime. You can return here any time you wish as you prepare for the birth. As you become relaxed, you'll remember this wonderfully serene place deep within you throughout the birth process.

"Enjoy this precious time 'meeting' your baby before she journeys through labour into your arms."

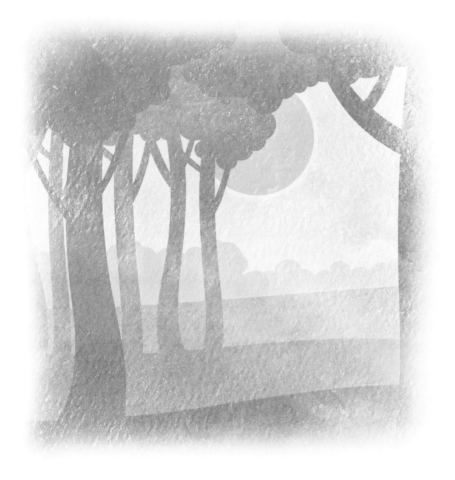

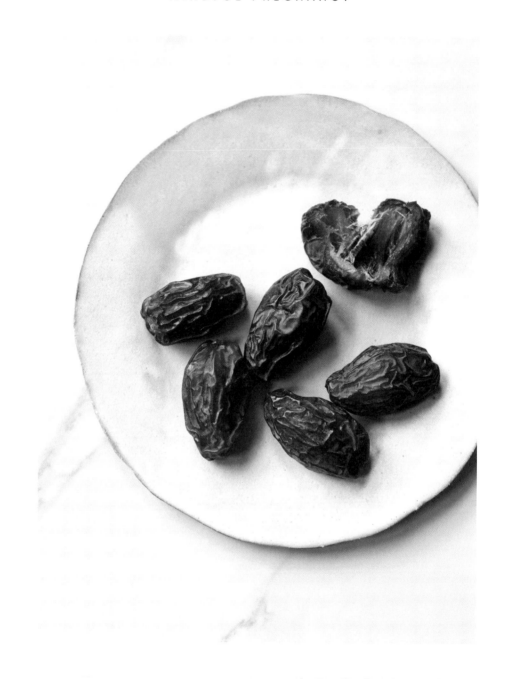

Medjool dates

Known as the fruit of the gods, dates have become the fruit for third trimester mums. Several studies suggest eating around six dates a day during the last four weeks of pregnancy can significantly benefit your labour.

In one study, the dilation stage of labour was significantly shorter in women who consumed **dates** compared to those who didn't. Plus 96 per cent of the women who ate dates went into spontaneous labour and didn't have to be induced. Women who consumed dates were also less likely to experience heavy bleeding after birth.

Dates are rich in minerals and fibre, but high in natural sugars, so be aware of this if you have gestational diabetes. Either eat dates straight from the bag, or if you find they are too sweet for you, add them to a tagine or stew, or stuff them with almonds or cream cheese for a nutritious snack. Alternatively, make **peanut date bites** by blending together 10 pitted dates and 150g of chopped unsalted roasted peanuts. When blitzed, form into small balls and enjoy.

Bond with your baby

*Intentionally sending loving thoughts to your baby
builds the bond with him long before he is in your arms.
You can do this meditation at any time and anywhere
– at the office, in a shop, while commuting, or at home.*

1

Place your hands on your belly. Close your eyes and take a few deep breaths as you connect with your baby. Notice any sounds around you and place all your attention on those sounds. Then bring your attention back to your breathing.

2

Move your attention to your body. Are you aware of any tension or heaviness? No need to change anything – just be present.

3

Do you notice any subtle movements from your baby? Imagine this is the first, special time you feel your baby move.

4

Smile as you send your baby loving thoughts – your baby safely cocooned, floating in love, appreciation, and joy.

5

Bring your focus back to the rise and fall of your breath, bringing oxygen, calm, and connectedness to you and your baby.

"Allow yourself to be present in this moment — just you and your baby lovingly connected as life races by."

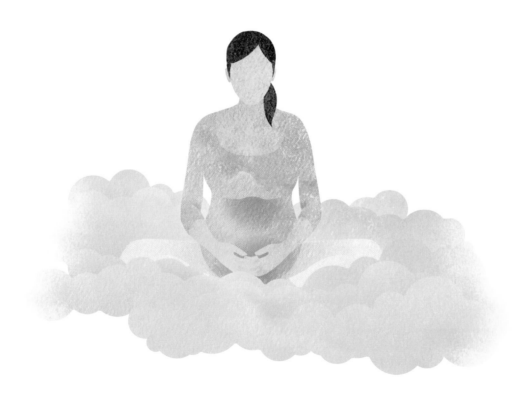

A special memory

Rehearse this exercise with your partner in the third trimester. Bring to mind a special memory, so during labour, when a surge begins, your partner can remind you of the memory and you can focus on that.

1

Think of a special time with your partner when you felt safe and comfortable. What were you doing? Were you on holiday?

2

Ask your partner to describe the scene to you, making the memories come alive and making you feel as if you are actually there. How do you feel? Your partner can prompt you using words such as "safe", "loved", "supported", "relaxed", "happy", or "excited".

3

What can you see? Blossom on a branch, the sun sparkling on a lake, an ice-capped mountain? Be there in that scene.

4

What can you hear? Soft music, waves, your partner's voice? What can you smell? Suntan lotion can be a powerful anchor.

5

Bask in all the memories, allowing your body to react to these positive, loving recollections as you finish the exercise.

"The more detail your partner can describe, the more effective this hypnobirthing exercise will be."

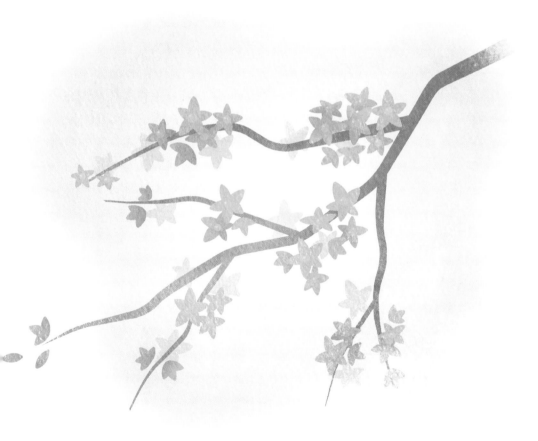

Practice and posture

In the third trimester your body continues to adapt as it creates space for your baby and gets ready for birth. Your yoga practice will be important as it increases your comfort levels and connection with your baby.

This can be a challenging trimester emotionally and physically as you get closer to the big day. Over the coming weeks, notice how mindful movement, anchored by your focused breathing, increases your confidence, excitement, strength, and mental stamina for labour and birth. Return "home" to your breath often, on or off the mat. This is a time of graciousness and generous acceptance as you prepare for mindful motherhood. Your yoga practice can be an incredibly profound way to continue connecting with your body and baby during the last weeks of pregnancy and as you journey through labour together.

"Continue with slow, intentional movement as you build strength and stamina for labour."

30-MINUTE SEQUENCE

As your due date grows closer, focused movement will calm your mind and body, while continuing to build strength and stamina. Always listen to your body, use props for extra stability, and break down the sequence if you wish.

01

MOUNTAIN POSE

It's easy to forget about the importance of posture in this trimester, so stand tall and strong, with your feet hip-distance apart and your arms by your sides. Ground your feet firmly and bring your pelvis to its neutral position. As you inhale, lengthen through your torso and elongate your neck. Hold for a few minutes.

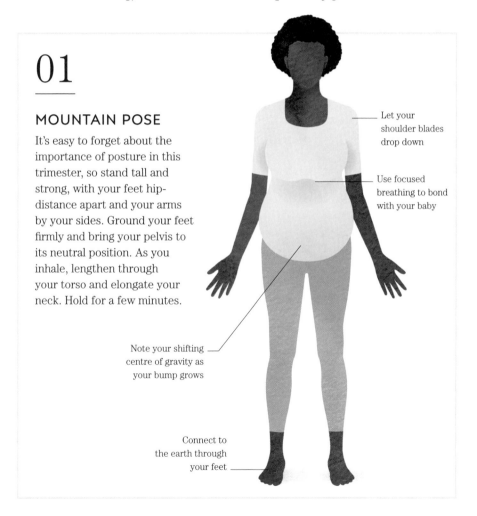

Let your shoulder blades drop down

Use focused breathing to bond with your baby

Note your shifting centre of gravity as your bump grows

Connect to the earth through your feet

02

SEATED WARRIOR

This modified Warrior Pose *(see p106)* uses a chair to help open the hips. Sit facing forwards on the edge of a sturdy chair, arms raised in a T shape. Turn your left foot out 90 degrees and, as you turn your body and head in the same direction, let your back leg straighten. Hold for a few breaths, then repeat on the other side.

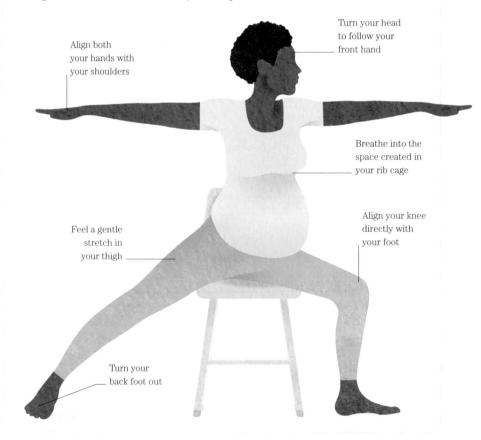

Align both
your hands with
your shoulders

Turn your head
to follow your
front hand

Breathe into the
space created in
your rib cage

Feel a gentle
stretch in
your thigh

Align your knee
directly with
your foot

Turn your
back foot out

03

LOW LUNGE

Deep, mindful stretches are important this trimester to improve blood circulation in the legs and reduce swelling. Come off the chair and into Tabletop. Move your left foot forwards next to your left hand. Slowly move your right leg back and breathe into the deep stretch of the hips and thighs. Press down into your fingertips or use blocks as you lift and open your chest. Hold for a minute, then come back to Tabletop and repeat on the other side.

SUPPLE HIPS

Tight hips in pregnancy can result in lower back discomfort, so use this pose, which helps with hip flexibility.

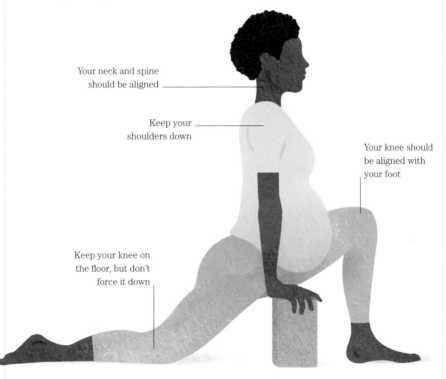

Your neck and spine should be aligned

Keep your shoulders down

Your knee should be aligned with your foot

Keep your knee on the floor, but don't force it down

04

SQUAT

Position blocks or blankets on your mat. With your feet wider than your hips, knees bent, lower yourself slowly onto the blocks. Put your hands together and use your elbows to gently stretch the inner thighs. Inhale, drawing up your pelvic floor. Exhale and relax your pelvic floor. Press into your heels to come out of the squat slowly. You can also do this against a wall for extra support.

PELVIC FLOOR STRENGTHENER

Squatting is a perfect exercise for the third trimester as it engages, lengthens, and strengthens the pelvic floor.

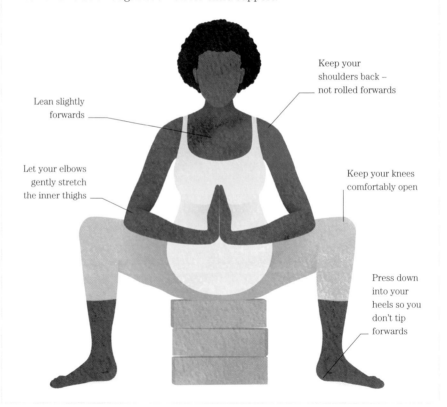

Lean slightly forwards

Keep your shoulders back – not rolled forwards

Let your elbows gently stretch the inner thighs

Keep your knees comfortably open

Press down into your heels so you don't tip forwards

05 TABLETOP

Slowly move to your hands and knees: knees apart, hands aligned under your shoulders. Engage your core so your back is flat. Hold for several breaths.

Let your shoulders sink down

Spread your fingers into a starfish shape

06 HIP CIRCLES

Gently move your pelvis backwards and then forwards in a clockwise motion. Repeat a few times, then move anticlockwise.

Move your pelvis back only to your comfort level

Engage your stomach muscles to hug your baby to you

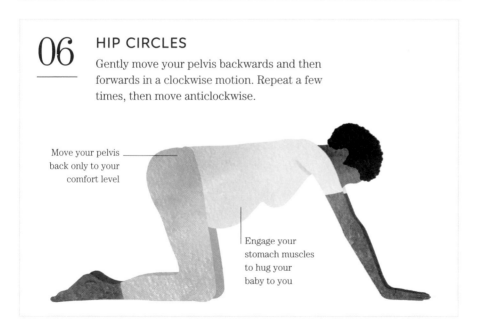

07 CAT

From Tabletop, exhale, lift your ribs, and arch your back like a cat. Hug your baby to you, practising slow, deep breathing, then return to Tabletop.

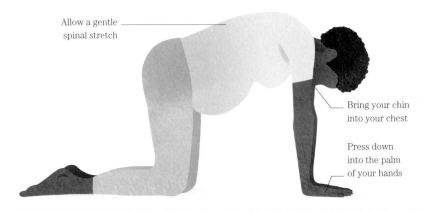

Allow a gentle spinal stretch

Bring your chin into your chest

Press down into the palm of your hands

08 COW

From Tabletop, imagine your heart is moving forwards so you don't drop your belly. Look up, keeping your neck and head aligned.

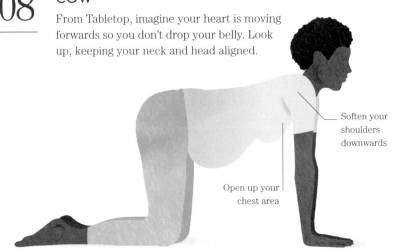

Soften your shoulders downwards

Open up your chest area

09

PUPPY POSE

From Cow, walk your hands towards the top of your mat, extend your arms, and lower your head to the mat. Open your knees wide enough to make space for your bump. Use a pillow to support your forehead and a bolster under your chest. If your wrists are sore, place your forearms on blocks. Hold this relaxing pose for up to a minute, calming your thoughts, then return to Tabletop.

OXYGEN BOOSTER

This pose brings oxygenated blood to all of the major organs of your body, including the uterus.

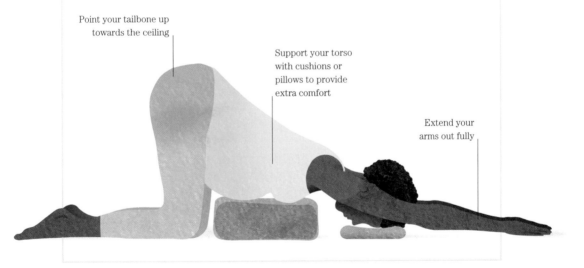

Point your tailbone up towards the ceiling

Support your torso with cushions or pillows to provide extra comfort

Extend your arms out fully

"Practise this pose to calm you when you feel anxious or worried."

149

10

HERO'S POSE

Kneel with a block or bolster under your pelvis and a rolled-up towel just above your ankles (over your Achilles tendon). Sit up tall, lengthening the spine. Stay in this position for several breaths, connecting with your baby, or for a short visualization.

RE-ENERGIZING

This pose stimulates the gut, reducing the risk of constipation and swelling of the legs, which are common issues during the third trimester.

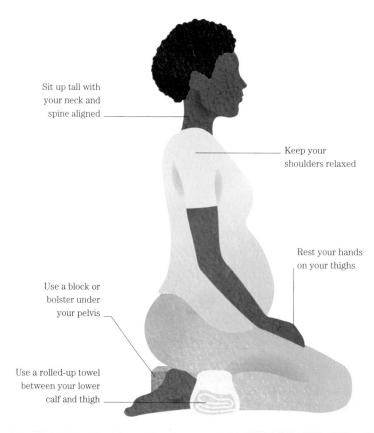

Sit up tall with your neck and spine aligned

Keep your shoulders relaxed

Rest your hands on your thighs

Use a block or bolster under your pelvis

Use a rolled-up towel between your lower calf and thigh

11 RECLINING HERO'S POSE

Deep breathing can be challenging in this trimester, but this pose allows for more spaciousness in the torso. Set up blocks and bolsters so you can lean back safely and comfortably. Supported by your hands, move slowly from Hero's Pose into a reclined position. Hold for several deep breaths, then drop your chin to your chest and walk your fingers forwards, back to Hero's Pose.

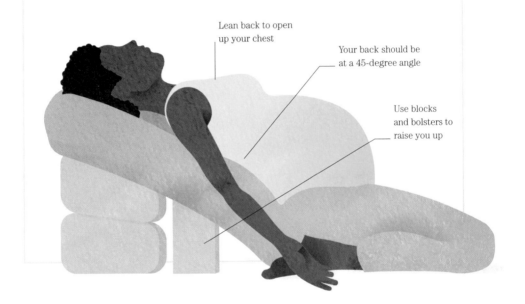

Lean back to open up your chest

Your back should be at a 45-degree angle

Use blocks and bolsters to raise you up

"This expansive, restorative pose promotes rest, reduces stress, and allows for mindful breathing."

12

SEATED PIGEON POSE

This pose helps to open up your hips, preparing you for labour. Sit up straight on a chair and roll your shoulders several times in both directions to release tension. Bring your right foot up and place it over your left thigh. Hold for 30 seconds for a comfortable stretch. Repeat with the left leg.

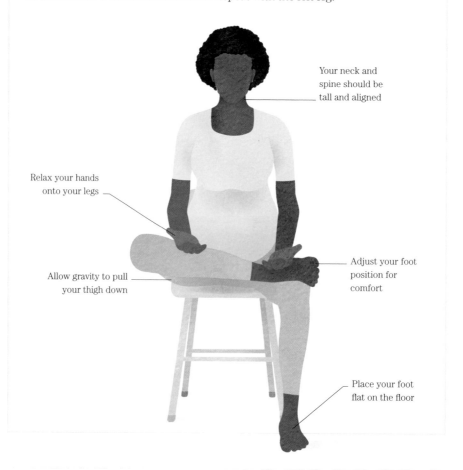

Your neck and spine should be tall and aligned

Relax your hands onto your legs

Allow gravity to pull your thigh down

Adjust your foot position for comfort

Place your foot flat on the floor

13

EASY POSE

Sit up tall facing straight ahead with your legs in front of you. Bend one leg until you can place your foot under the opposite thigh, then repeat with the other leg. Rest your hands on your belly. Close your eyes and hold for a few minutes. Inhale calm and exhale worry.

EXTRA SUPPORT

Practise this cross-legged pose against a wall, and place blocks or cushions under your knees and hips to support them fully.

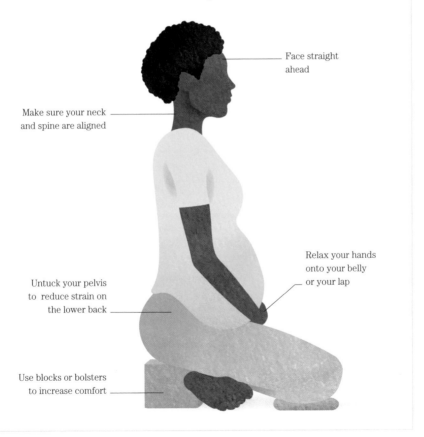

Face straight ahead

Make sure your neck and spine are aligned

Relax your hands onto your belly or your lap

Untuck your pelvis to reduce strain on the lower back

Use blocks or bolsters to increase comfort

14

BUTTERFLY

DEEP BREATHS

This soothing pose gives extra space to breathe deeply as your belly grows, and also triggers the relaxation response.

Sit on a folded blanket. Keep your back tall with your legs out in front of you. Slowly bend your knees, hold the soles of your feet together and bring them in towards you. Allow your legs to gently flap like butterfly wings for a few breaths. Notice the stretch in your legs. Relax your knees for a couple of breaths and press down again comfortably. Repeat several times.

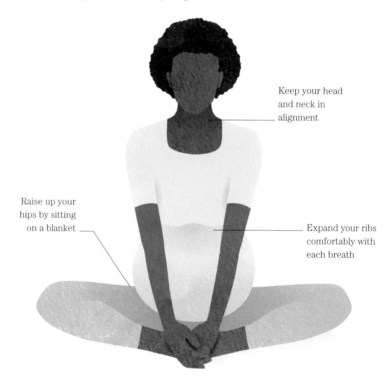

Keep your head and neck in alignment

Raise up your hips by sitting on a blanket

Expand your ribs comfortably with each breath

15

COBBLER'S POSE

From Butterfly, move your feet out slightly so your legs form a diamond shape. Lean forwards and walk your hands out past your feet to stretch your lower back and buttocks, but do not lean on your bump. Hold for a few breaths, then slowly walk your hands back, pulling your feet in closer, and flap your butterfly wings several times. This pose helps to reduce fatigue.

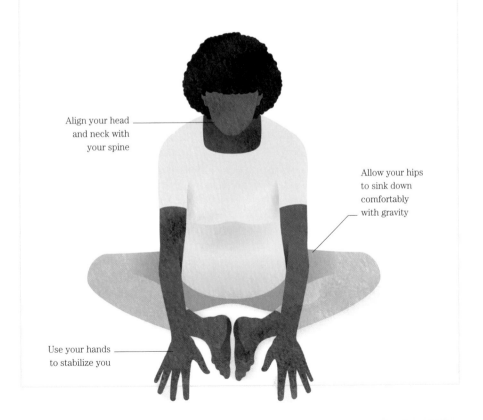

Align your head and neck with your spine

Allow your hips to sink down comfortably with gravity

Use your hands to stabilize you

CALMING
STRETCH

Some anxiety is normal
as labour approaches, but
deep restorative breaths in
this pose will calm an
overactive mind.

16

SEATED SIDE STRETCH

Side-stretching poses are great in the third trimester
to lengthen the muscles between the ribs and pelvis,
helping with breathing. From Cobbler's Pose, cross your
legs and support your hips and legs with cushions if you
wish. Raise your right hand over your head and slowly
lean into a side stretch. Bend your elbow and place
your left palm on the floor or on a block. Move to your
comfort level and hold for several restorative breaths.
Repeat on the other side.

Take care not to
lean forwards

Feel a deep
stretch in the side
of your abdomen

Lean into your
supporting hand
and elbow

17

SIDE-LYING RESTING POSE

Lie down on your left-hand side and place a pillow under your head. Straighten your bottom leg, place another pillow or blankets between your legs, and shift your top leg forwards. Focus on your breathing or on a visualization. Notice how your baby may move as you calm your body and mind. Stay here for about 10 minutes, mindfully scanning your body to release tension, then sit up gradually, before slowly moving to standing so you don't feel faint.

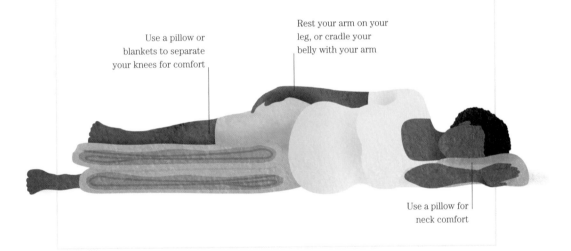

Use a pillow or blankets to separate your knees for comfort

Rest your arm on your leg, or cradle your belly with your arm

Use a pillow for neck comfort

"Come out of this pose slowly to avoid the risk of dizziness."

YOUR LABOUR AND BIRTH

*Your baby is waiting to meet you!
Labour and birth can seem daunting, and
it's natural to have concerns. However,
there are ways to stack the odds in your
favour of having the birth of your dreams,
by using visualization, hypnobirthing,
breathing techniques, optimal labour
positions, and essential oils.*

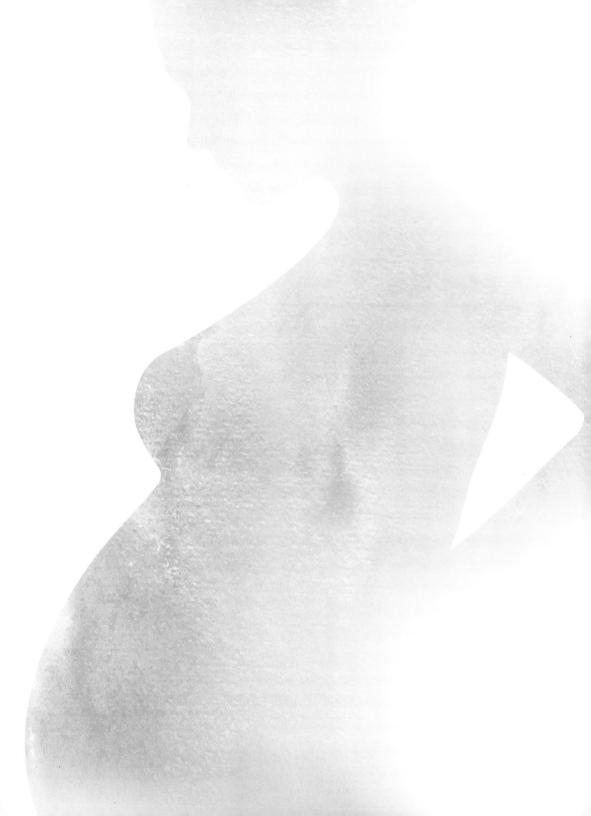

Your labour and birth

A mindful approach to labour and birth is a flexible one so you can meet your baby with joy. Using these positive practices will give you the strength and resilience to have an empowered birth experience.

Read through this chapter in the weeks before you are due to give birth so you can consider all the mindful strategies available to you. Try some of the exercises so you can see what you think will work best for you – this chapter is organized so the exercises follow the stages of your labour.

The way you think about pain changes how you experience the sensations of labour. The brain interprets those sensations based on your emotions, experience, culture, and expectations. Your thoughts can intensify those sensations or reduce them. A mindful approach to labour and pain means you do not resist the sensations of labour, which just causes more pain, but you approach them with an open and curious attitude. "I want this" can be a great mantra in labour.

"*Labour is like an intricate dance, where your baby is your partner and the choreographer.*"

Notice the places in your body where you feel the sensations the most … can you allow those sensations to rise and fall like the ocean? Each wave is a little different, and each wave will require you to draw on your instincts, encouraging you to move your body in a certain way, or to breathe more deeply. When you listen mindfully to what's happening in your body, you can hear what your baby is asking of you.

In the event that an unexpected complication arises, this mindful preparation for birth will significantly improve your experience during labour and your recovery afterwards.

An undisturbed birth

To optimize labour hormones and your natural pain-relieving brain chemicals, such as oxytocin, there are certain conditions that must be met. Birth experts refer to this as an "undisturbed" birth. Like other mammals, we need privacy, warmth, dim lighting, and feelings of safety and support so we can turn off our "thinking" brain and allow our instincts to take over.

When the conditions of an undisturbed birth are provided for a labouring mum, her progress is likely to be quicker and less painful. Anxiety and stress cause the brain to release

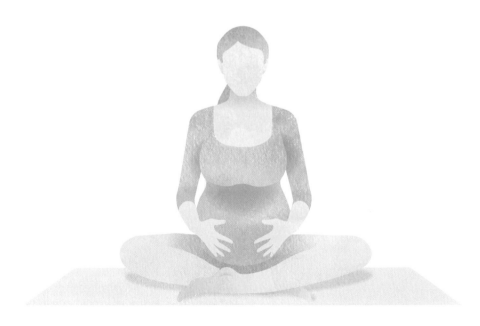

adrenaline, which blocks oxytocin, so the calmer you are in labour, the less painful your labour is likely to be.

Working with labour sensations

Have you ever banged your elbow and then rubbed it quickly? By rubbing it, you created a competing sensation that reached a neurological "gate" in the spine and closed the gate, reducing your pain perception. Massage during labour, a water birth, and a TENS machine all use this "gating" system of pain perception to compete with the pain signals of labour.

Meditation (*see p166, p170,* and *p176*), focused breathing (*see p172* and *p178*), hypnobirthing techniques, and soothing music can also all reduce pain during labour.

Using medication

There are many effective ways to manage labour sensations naturally (*see opposite*), but if you find you need additional support with medication, such as entonox (gas or air), pethidine, diamorphine, remifentanil, or an epidural, allow yourself the grace to make that choice without guilt. A mindful pregnancy becomes a mindful labour when you are compassionate towards the unfolding experience.

A mindful caesarean

A caesarean birth involves major abdominal surgery, but for a small number of mothers this is the safest option. A caesarean can still be a mindful experience, especially if it's a planned one. Explore some birth preferences with your health-care provider that can make a clinical, medical experience into a more family-centred celebration of your baby's arrival.

The first stage of labour

This is usually the longest stage, especially for a first-time mother. Your cervix is thinning and you begin to dilate. Mindfully conserving your energy will be important in the early stages. Gentle yoga stretches, slow breathing, and hypnobirthing facilitate the optimal hormone release to progress your labour naturally as you and your baby journey together.

The second stage of labour

This is the pushing stage, when your body starts to nudge your baby along the birth canal. Although many mums feel quite tired at this point, your body naturally releases adrenaline to give you an energy boost. This stage of labour is usually accompanied by

MINDFUL COMFORT MEASURES

As the sensations of labour become more powerful, instinctual movements will direct you to comfort strategies that support the physiology of birth – see below for some of the main strategies.

Using a pool/bath

This is one of the most effective comfort measures for labour as it increases your natural oxytocin significantly, and shortens labour.

Movement

Yoga (*see pp182–9*), walking, dancing – any kind of instinctive movement reduces pain. Let your body and baby lead the way.

Acupressure and massage

Firm massage to the back and hips can feel magical during labour, while acupressure can increase your comfort.

Doula

A doula is a professional birth companion who provides you with emotional support and focus throughout your labour and birth.

TENS machine

A TENS machine is a small, portable device that emits low-voltage currents and is used for pain relief in labour. The brain pays attention to the tingle from the TENS machine, which shuts the gate to other sensations coming from the uterus that may be causing you pain.

Rebozo

You can use a rebozo (a long, woven scarf) during labour to gently lift your belly as you remain on all fours. This relaxes the abdominal muscles and uterine ligaments to give your baby space to move into the optimal position, and also feels wonderful for your lower back. Or you can cover your head and your birth partner's to create a "cave", allowing the world to disappear as you and your birth partner breathe together.

»

feelings of intense and almost irresistible pressure rather than pain, as your body begins the final stage before you meet your baby.

The length of this stage can be influenced by your position *(see p183)*, your baby's position, and the use of an epidural, which may make this stage longer. If you are mobile, your midwife can help you into a supported squat *(see p188)*, all fours *(see p189)*, or side-lying position *(see p189)*.

Your midwife will remind you to try not to push as your baby's head is starting to crown so the emergence of your baby's head can be as slow and controlled as possible. You may be encouraged to pant or blow like you're gently blowing out a candle to help you to stay focused during these brief few moments *(see p178)*.

Mother-led mindful pushing rather than coached, cheerleading-style pushing is beneficial to you and your baby as you are following cues from your body to bear down at the right time instead of holding your breath for long periods. When tuned into the sensations of your body, you may instinctively move your legs closer together as your baby's head emerges.

Mindfully meeting your baby

The birth room can get very busy, so when you're getting close to the moment of birth, your birth partner

SKIN-TO-SKIN

You and your baby will significantly benefit from being kept together skin-to-skin in a quiet "golden hour" of bonding.

Benefits for you

Holding your baby skin-to-skin after birth can help to promote bonding with your newborn. It also facilitates breastfeeding and can reduce the risk of excessive bleeding after birth.

Benefits for your baby

Keeping your baby skin-to-skin can help regulate your baby's breathing, temperature, blood sugars, and stress response. It will also expose her to healthy bacteria, which will "seed" your baby's gut microbiome.

"There can be many different emotions when you meet your baby – allow space for all of them."

may want to ask for quiet in the room. You can also ask for a deliberate "pause" once your baby is placed skin-to-skin with you. During this time the cord can be left unclamped as you meet your baby, and you can listen to a specially chosen piece of music, or your birth partner can read a poem or prayer to celebrate the arrival of your baby.

The third stage of labour

During this stage the placenta and membrane are delivered. Talk to your midwife about your options based on your individual experience: if you've had a mindful birth and all is well, a natural third stage makes sense as you bask in oxytocin and endorphins, drinking in these precious moments.

In some cultures the cord is not clamped at all if parents choose an intact birth – allowing the placenta to stay attached to the baby for a little while after birth. The cutting of the cord symbolizes the end of your pregnancy, and for some parents, taking time to recognize and reflect on this symbolic moment is important.

Alternatively, you can choose a lotus birth, where the placenta stays attached to your baby for several days until the cord dries and naturally separates. In this case the placenta will need to be professionally treated with herbs as it is an organ that you'll carry with your baby for a few days.

The "golden hour"

The first hour after birth is a neurologically sensitive time for bonding, with massive brain activity in both mother and baby. During this quiet, undisturbed time, cuddle your baby skin-to-skin (*see opposite*). Your baby may instinctively find your breast and latch on, and all routine checks can be postponed until after your baby has had her first feed.

Meditation for labour

During labour use this meditation to focus on your breathing, helping you to soothe your mind and body. Practising this when you have any discomfort in pregnancy will help you to use it to best effect in labour.

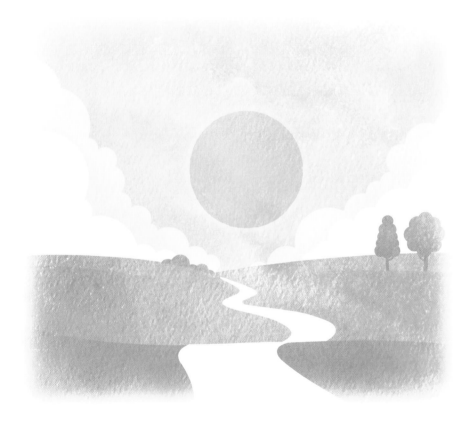

1

As the twinges start, remember that today you will meet your baby. Your mind, body, and baby are working together as your pregnancy ends and you continue the sacred journey into motherhood. Embrace your experience with appreciation and patience. Connect with the courage of the long lineage of birthing mothers who came before you.

2

Your breath will anchor you. Place your attention on your breathing. If your mind wanders, refocus it back to your breath.

3

Notice how the sensations in your uterus will rise, peak, and pass – every peak bringing you one step closer to meeting your baby. Allow deep belly breathing to soothe your labouring mind and body.

4

Are there other sensations occurring in your body? Allow yourself to be curious and kind about how your body is responding to your labour. If your response is to tense parts of your body, can you relax those areas?

5

Notice what is happening emotionally between your surges as you rest. Does your mind wander to scenes of joy or worry? Stay with your baby as you journey together. As the next surge begins, deepen your focus and breathing and with kind awareness, send loving thoughts to your baby and appreciation to your body as your journey continues. All is well.

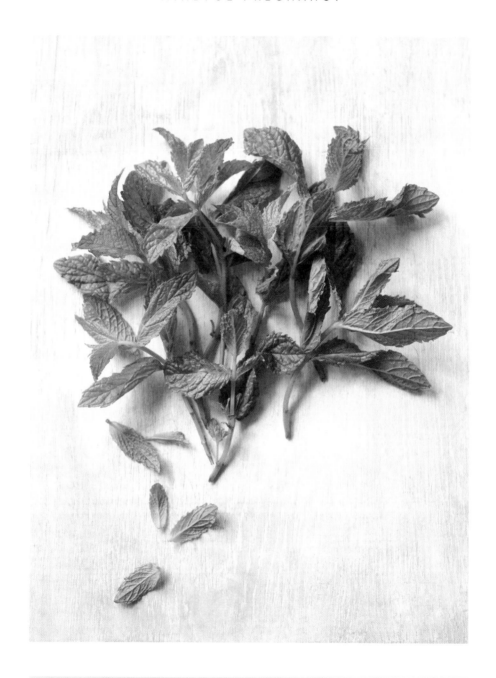

Essential oils for labour

Choose an oil or oils that facilitate emotional relaxation but also help with focus and stamina. In labour, use one or two drops on a tissue that you or your birth partner can hold, so you can discard it if it's overwhelming.

Research suggests when **lavender** is used during labour women have less pain and nausea and it can help to reduce anxiety. **Jasmine** can help relieve pain, and **frankincense** encourages deep, slow breathing. As labour progresses and you feel the need to mobilize, **citrus oils** such as **lemon** and **orange** can be stimulating. If it feels like you can't manage those last pushes, then **peppermint** oil is ideal as it increases focus. As your baby's sense of smell is heightened right after birth to facilitate bonding with you, use just a few drops of peppermint oil on a tissue or cotton wool ball and discard before your baby arrives.

"Peppermint is a wonderfully refreshing oil that boosts stamina."

Power thoughts for labour

Before you go into labour it can be helpful to choose a word or words to focus your mind on during a surge. The more you can make the word or words your own, the more effective and calming they will be.

Yes

I want this. I mindfully and joyfully accept our path together.

Breathe

I breathe in loving energy and courage and breathe out worry.

Yield

My cervix melts and yields to my baby's gentle arrival.

Open

My mind and body open to birth.

"Find words that naturally resonate with you. Try each of these words and notice how they make your body feel."

Soften

Everything is softening
as my baby journeys
to my arms.

Release

I release all mental
and physical tension.

Allow

I allow my baby to lead the way.
I allow all emotions.

Welcome

I welcome the sensations
bringing my baby
to me.

Using the "O" sound

As you move deeper into labour, one of the most effective ways to reduce stress and pain is by mindful breathing. By adding vocalization you are also using meditative sound as a way to relax your body and stay grounded.

1

Place your hand at the bottom of your throat, where your chest and throat meet.

2

Breathe deeply and as you exhale make the "O" sound – it can be as loud as you like. Let the sound continue while you release your breath completely. Make sure that your jaw and throat are relaxed. Many midwives believe there is a strong link between a relaxed jaw and a relaxed pelvic floor.

3

Notice the vibrations in your chest and hand as you make the "O" sound.

4

Experiment with different low sounds such as "Ahhhhh", "Hmmm", and "Ohhhhhh".

5

Try the sounds at different pitches to see what feels best for you as your labour progresses.

"When vocalizing, imagine the 'O' as an ever-widening circle representing the opening of the cervix."

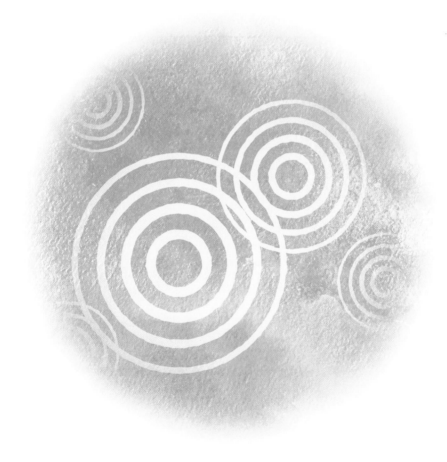

Homeopathic remedies for labour

Homeopathic practitioners advise taking remedies before and during labour to help alleviate any emotional challenges, such as worry or lack of confidence, as well as any physical ones, such as tiredness or backache.

There are a number of homeopathic remedies you can take, and different remedies may be needed or combined depending on how your labour progresses. According to the British Homeopathic Association, taking **Arnica montana** during labour will minimize bruising and bleeding. **Aconitum** is advised for fear and anxiety during labour especially if the surges are very close together; and **Chamomilla** is recommended for slow dilation and backache in labour.

"As homeopathic remedies come in various potencies, see a homeopath for a remedy specifically for you."

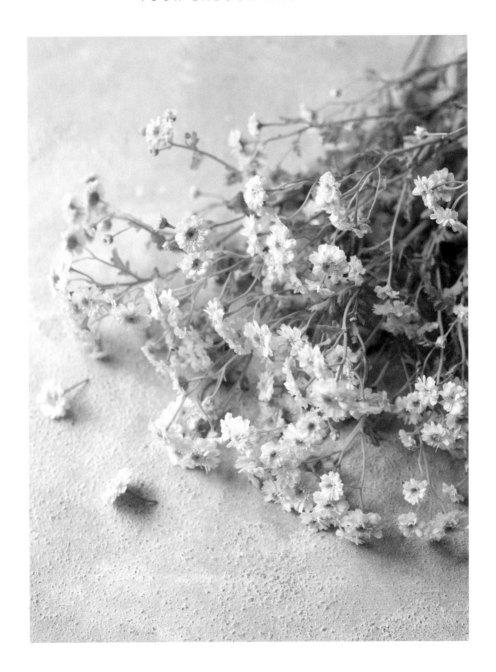

The lotus flower

The opening flower is a universal metaphor for birth and combines the elements of unfolding, ease, and softness. Use this imagery during labour or as part of your daily mental preparation for birth from 37 weeks.

1

Sit or lie down – whichever is most comfortable. Close your eyes and simply focus your attention on your breathing.

2

Bring to mind either the image of the lotus flower or your favourite flower. Thinking of the scent makes this imagery even more effective.

3

If your attention wanders simply guide your mind back to that imagery, or any imagery that suggests gentle opening and expansion.

4

Visualize the delicate flower petals opening one by one slowly and easily.

5

As your uterus surges gently and easily with each petal opening, your body also unfolds with ease and grace. Imagine your heart is also opening and expanding with each inhalation – your heart has an unlimited capacity of love for your new baby and the experiences ahead.

"*A flower opening is a very powerful visualization you can use during labour.*"

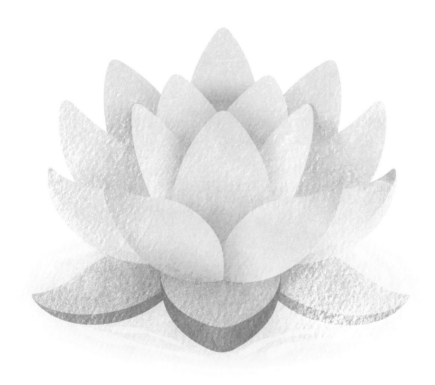

Breathing for pushing

Slow, controlled breathing is essential for this stage of labour to increase the flow of rich blood to you and your baby. Allow your body to find the most productive, comfortable position when you need to push.

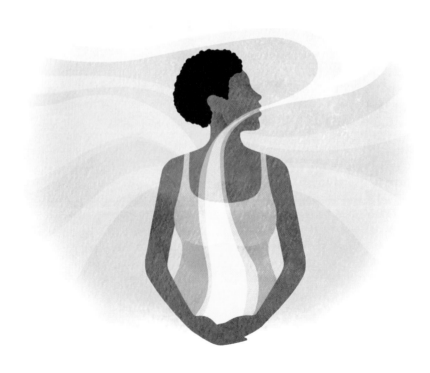

"Follow the natural rhythms of your body and trust that the knowledge of how to push is already within you."

1

Welcome each wave as it strengthens. Keep your jaw relaxed and your throat open as you inhale and exhale mindfully.

2

Let your breaths deepen as the pressure builds up and the urge to push becomes irresistible. Focus on long, deep breaths as your body starts to nudge your baby along the birth canal. Try not to hold your breath as this reduces oxygen to you and your baby. Grunting and deep, low vocalizing may help.

3

When your baby's head is about to be born, focus on slow, deep breaths. Try panting or blowing like you're gently blowing out a candle. The intensity of these sensations can feel overwhelming, so keeping all of your focus on your breathing will help you to feel calmer and more in control.

4

Once your baby's head has been born, make loud sighs with a relaxed jaw to bring your new baby into your arms.

Meeting your baby

When the physical work of labour is done, your mind needs time to pause and appreciate the precious first minutes with your baby. Those fleeting moments will be etched into your heart and mind forever.

1

Mentally create a cocoon of calm or a birth bubble for you and your baby as you finally "meet" on the outside.

2

With feelings of joy, relief, and awe gather your baby to you and lie her skin-to-skin on your warm chest.

3

Breathe in the scent of your new baby and allow her to rest in the nest of your loving embrace after her long journey.

4

Softly speak words of love and whisper wellness into her ear – your baby is listening. She recognizes your voice – she too has been waiting for this moment. As every mother before you has done, instinctively explore every finger and toe in awe. You absorb her presence – and she yours.

5

With humility, mindful intention, and deep appreciation for the precious gift of parenthood, welcome your new baby.

"Take in your baby and appreciate the monumental transformation that has just occurred for you both."

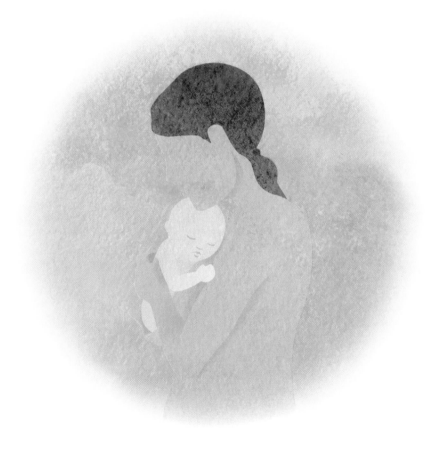

Labour and birth

Using yoga as mindful movement in labour can provide a deep reservoir of comfort, calmness, and confidence. In addition, women who change positions frequently in labour often experience shorter, more comfortable births.

Your labour is a unique journey unlike any other. As you move through the different sensations of labour some positions will naturally feel more comforting. Try the poses on pages 183–9 to see which feel best as you progress through your labour, and allow your body's wisdom to guide you as you seek out the best positions when resting or experiencing twinges or surges. Throughout your pregnancy you have been cultivating a deep, mindful connection with your breath, body, and baby to anchor you during any challenging moments in birth and beyond, so allow your body and baby to lead the way to intuitive movements as you connect with your inner strength.

"You are connected in courage with thousands of mothers around the world also giving birth today."

ACTIVE POSES FOR LABOUR

In early labour choose positions and activities that promote rest and energy conservation. As labour progresses, your mindful connection to your body will intuitively direct you to optimal upright positions to facilitate your baby's birth.

FIGURE OF EIGHT ON A BIRTHING BALL

The birthing ball is well known as a way to reduce discomfort in active labour and create more space in your pelvis. Sit on the ball, your feet on the floor, and lean forwards slightly until you find a comfortable position. Move your hips in a clockwise motion, making a figure of eight, then change direction.

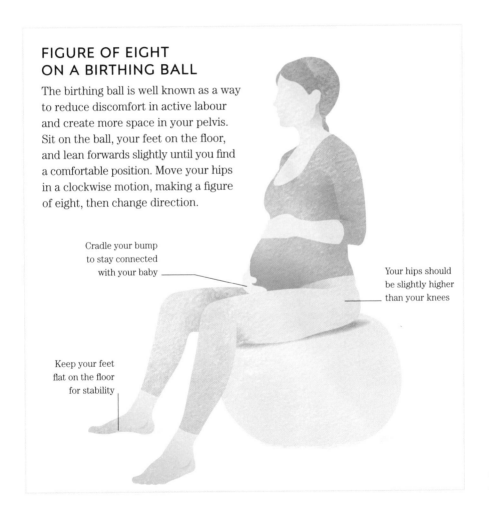

Cradle your bump to stay connected with your baby

Your hips should be slightly higher than your knees

Keep your feet flat on the floor for stability

SUPPORTED SQUAT

Squatting on a birthing stool with your birth partner behind you for support will comfort you and takes some of the effort out of the position so you can stay present with focused breathing.

>> *See page 146*

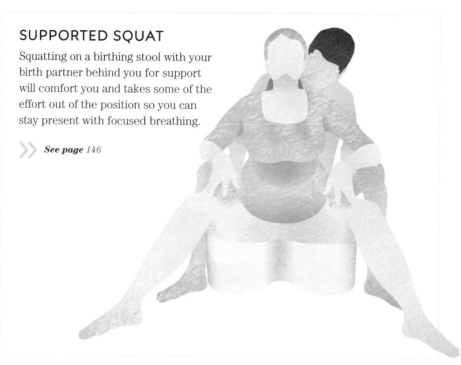

TABLETOP WITH HIP ROLLS

This position takes the pressure off the lower back as gravity pulls your baby towards the front of the pelvis. You'll find rolling your hips brings instant comfort.

>> *See page 147*

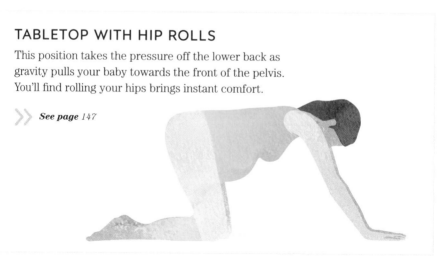

"Play soothing music to support your instinctive movements."

CAT

This is a great pose for active labour as it allows the pelvis to expand and open as your baby moves through it. It also releases tension in the shoulders and neck.

>> ***See page*** *148*

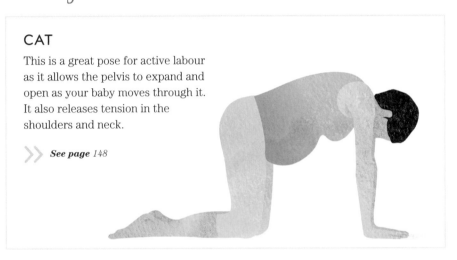

COW

This position on all fours is fabulous for the release of lower back tension and discomfort. You can be either on the floor or the bed, depending on your preference.

>> ***See page*** *148*

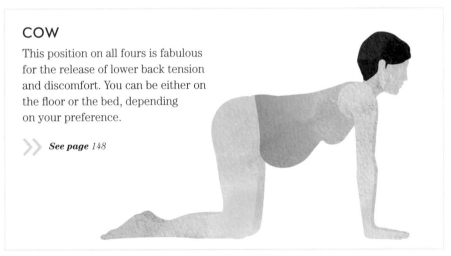

RESTING POSES IN LABOUR

Early labour is a time for resting, both mentally and physically, to conserve energy for the work ahead. Experiment with these poses to see which are the most nurturing and restful, or try Side-lying Pose (see p157).

EASY POSE

Easy Pose is the perfect position to rest in and practise your hypnobirthing or meditation exercises with a quiet alertness. Use props to support your body.

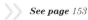 ***See page** 153*

MOUNTAIN POSE

Mountain Pose can help you feel grounded and centred during labour as you use your breath to connect with the earth.

***See page** 143*

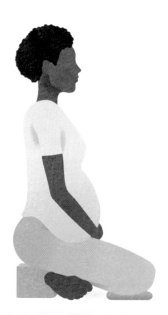

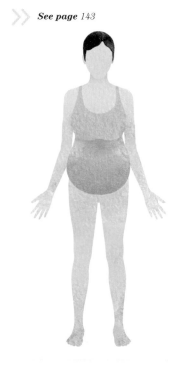

BUTTERFLY

In this variation of Easy Pose (*see opposite*) bring the soles of your feet together firmly to activate the solar plexus reflexology pressure point to calm and ground you.

》》 **See page** *154*

See page *154*

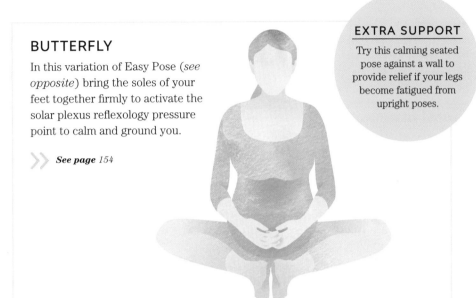

EXTRA SUPPORT

Try this calming seated pose against a wall to provide relief if your legs become fatigued from upright poses.

CHILD'S POSE

Child's Pose is a lovely way to help release the ligaments and muscles surrounding the uterus, giving your baby more room while inducing a state of relaxation and calm.

》》 **See page** *114*

See page *114*

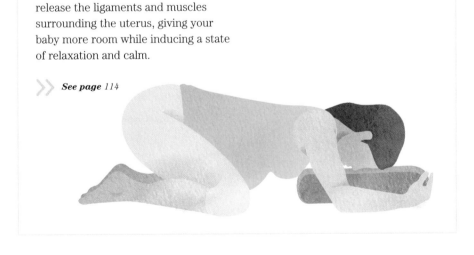

BIRTHING POSITIONS

*As the moment of birth approaches, the sensations of intense
pressure deep in the pelvis drive mothers to adopt positions
that work with gravity and physiology. For a short time your
surges may lengthen as your body nudges your baby along.*

SUPPORTED SQUAT

When squatting in labour, gravity
will help to bring your baby to you.
If you find squatting unassisted is
a challenge, sit on a birthing stool
and let your birth partner support
most of your weight to take the
pressure off your legs.

>> *See page 146*

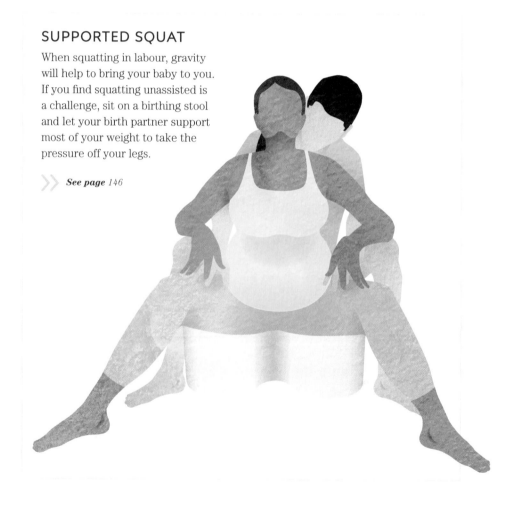

TABLETOP

If you have an urge to push before you are fully
dilated you can move down onto your elbows and
take the pressure off the cervix. Between surges,
move from Tabletop back into Child's Pose.

>> **See page** *147*

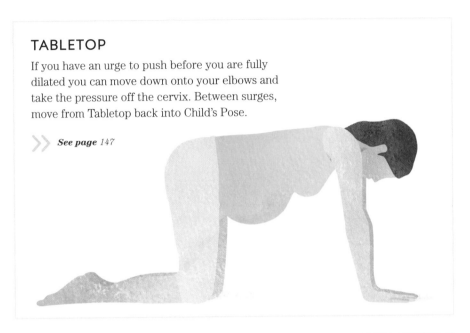

SIDE-LYING RESTING POSE

If you've had a long labour and are too tired to remain
upright, a side-lying position can be a welcome respite.
Your midwife can support your top leg during pushing
and you can rest and recharge between surges.

>> **See page** *157*

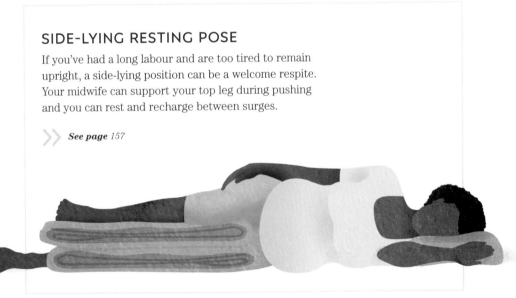

YOU AND YOUR BABY

As you settle in with your new baby, there are many ways to optimize your physical recovery mindfully. Here you'll find natural remedies for post-birth healing and improved sleep, as well as nutritional advice to promote a healthy milk supply. During this time of intense emotional adjustment, meditation and breathing exercises will anchor you as you adjust to life as a new mother.

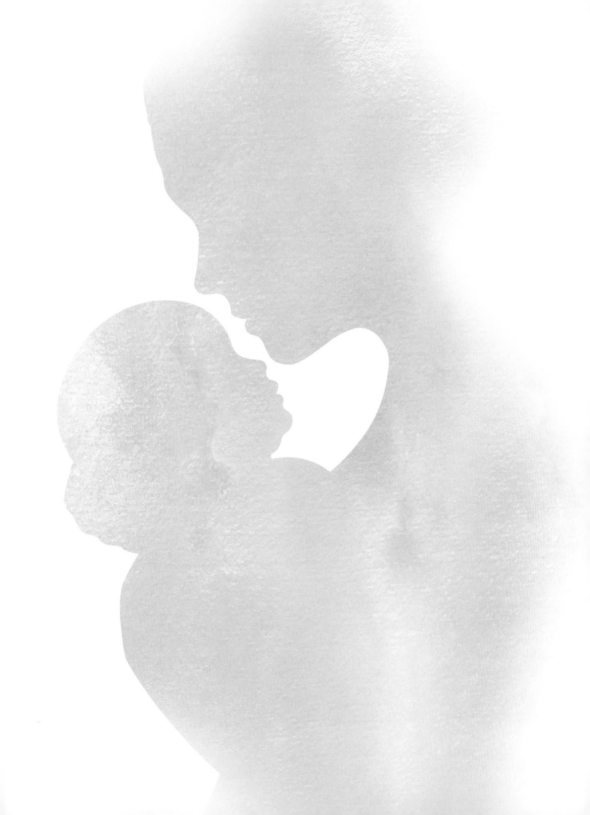

You and your baby

Not only has your baby been born, but you, too, have been born as a mother. Be gentle with yourself and accepting of your emotions as you get to know your baby and adapt to your new role.

Bonding with your baby

Although many mothers feel a huge rush of love for their newborn immediately after birth, this isn't the case for all mums, especially after a difficult birth. Remember that bonding with your baby happens over a lifetime – not just in the first hour after birth.

Becoming a mindful mother

Mindful mothering is a natural extension of a mindful pregnancy. It is a gentle, curious, and accepting approach to being a new mum that is abundantly generous in kindness.

Being mindful is a lot easier when everything is rosy. During challenging times, for example when you're sleep deprived, your mindful awareness will be even more important. Notice how you talk to yourself about your abilities as a mother and how your thoughts impact your parenting, breastfeeding, and your connection with your baby. Even a moment of slow, focused breathing as you mindfully change your baby's nappy will help you stay present and connected with your baby.

When you are accepting and kind towards yourself without judgment, your capacity for the most fulfilling, flourishing relationship with yourself as a newly born mother and your beautiful new baby is limitless.

Managing emotions

This is a season in your life of intense physical and emotional changes that will alter every day. Some days it may feel like a season of storms, and other days will feel sunny and fresh. The storms always pass and so will the intensity of this season of your life. In the first days after birth your hormones are likely to be in free fall, and it's normal to feel tired and tearful. Remind yourself that this is just temporary. Both you and your partner can benefit from mindful breathing *(see p196 and p210)* to help you navigate intense emotions, especially if you are feeling overwhelmed.

Soothing remedies

As your volume of milk starts to come in a few days after birth you may experience swollen, hard, and hot breasts. Frequent feeding can help with engorgement, and cold cabbage leaves placed on the breast can be very soothing *(see p200)*.

Using a padsicle *(see p212)* or taking a herbal bath (but not until a few days after the birth, *see p212*) can help to reduce any perineal tenderness.

Skin-to-skin settling

Often a newborn baby will have their first feed and then sleep for a few hours. However, on the second night your newborn is likely to be active, unsettled, and hungry. This is normal newborn behaviour and keeping your baby skin-to-skin may help him settle.

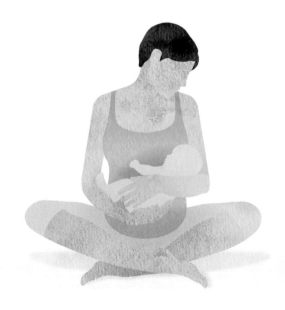

Re-energize

Taking even just a few minutes to meditate every day can restore and recharge your mind and body as a new mother and help you to feel refreshed and ready for what each moment brings.

1

Allow your mind to become quiet and your muscles to relax, from your head to your toes. Feel more comfortable with each passing moment.

2

Notice areas where your muscles are tense and let the feeling of relaxation begin there. The gentle rise and fall of your chest is so calming – each time you breathe out, your chest lowers gently and you feel as if all the tension is leaving your body. As you breathe in, feel yourself becoming even more deeply relaxed. Just rest…

3

Use visualization to focus your mind and provide a mental holiday for a few moments. Imagine a peaceful place: a quiet cabin in the mountains, a calm lake, a forest where you listen to the sounds of nature. Imagine yourself there now, relaxing in this peaceful place. Bring up all the details in your mind, drifting in this beautiful, calm place. Feel yourself relaxing even more deeply.

4

You are floating like a feather down through the air, moving from side to side, and drifting even deeper now. Your arms and legs are so heavy. You're sinking down as if surrounded by pillows. Sinking deeper and deeper into calm and comfort. Sinking into softness. Surrounded by softness. Resting…

5

You are feeling rested and restored, ready for any challenge. This time is well spent. Your wellbeing matters.

You are enough

As a new parent, life can feel isolating at times. Practise this exercise regularly so that you have the headspace to recognize what's going on in your mind and make friends with even the most difficult emotions.

1

Sit comfortably and focus on your breathing. Move your awareness from the top of your head down to your feet. Breathe in self-compassion and breathe out self-doubt. When ready, think of a difficulty that is bringing up challenging emotions. Notice how you may be inclined to push away those emotions.

2

Imagine a loving, wise figure representing unconditional love and nurturing, enveloping you in a warm blanket of love.

3

Allow this wise figure to support you as you hear these words: "Everything will be okay. You are enough. You are not alone."

4

This compassionate figure is always with you – it is a sacred part of you. You can connect with this part of you at any time.

5

Bring attention to your breath and allow this wise part of you to emerge and expand in the presence of challenging emotions.

"The more you can flow with the highs and lows, the more clarity and peace you can bring to each moment."

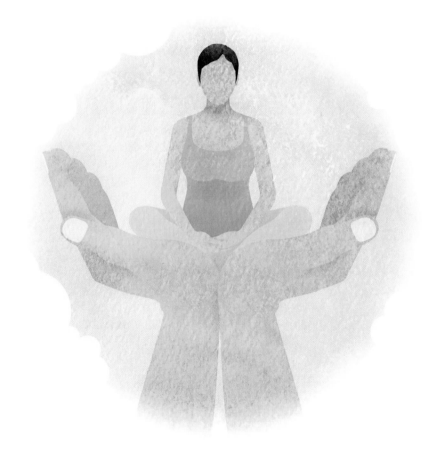

Nurturing postpartum foods

This is a time for self-care as much as baby care, so cultivate a compassionate, nurturing attitude towards yourself, starting with the foods you eat. Choose fresh, natural, energy providing and mood-boosting foods.

Make sure you are drinking plenty of water and are well hydrated, especially if breastfeeding. Good ideas for nourishing meals include replenishing, warming casseroles and stews, which can be packed with **vegetables** and **pulses**. Healthy, low-mercury fish such as **wild-caught salmon** and **sardines** contain "good" fats and can be served with a selection of **leafy green vegetables**. Include collagen- and protein-rich foods for tissue repair, such as **bone broth**. Also consider taking **probiotics** to support your immune system.

Before your baby arrives, stock up your freezer with pre-made dinners so it requires little effort to eat nutrient-dense, comfort food. Keep a selection of healthy snacks handy rather than sugar- or fat-laden ones that provide minimal nutrients. Foods containing **oats** are great for milk production *(see p205)* and can help to alleviate constipation.

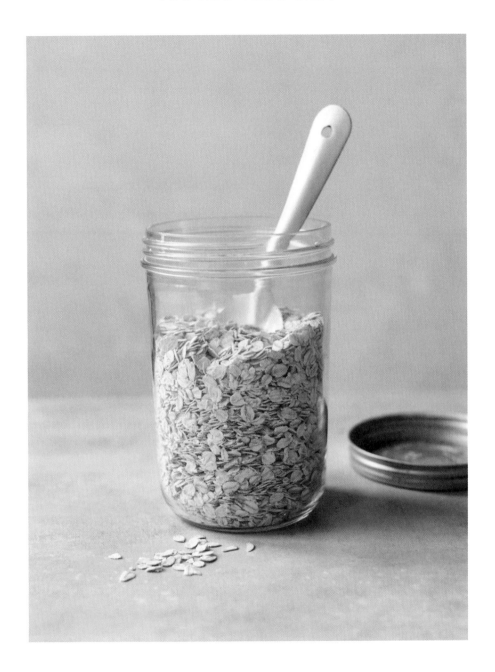

Cabbage leaves for engorgement

It's very common a few days after birth to find your breasts become uncomfortably heavy, hard, and even painful as your milk comes in fully. Cold, soothing cabbage leaves can help to relieve the engorgement.

The best way to help reduce engorgement is to keep your baby skin-to-skin over those first few days and cue feed often. Also ask your midwife about reverse pressure softening to ensure your baby can latch on well if you do become engorged. Applying **cabbage leaf compresses** to the breast can be very soothing and cooling and can help to reduce engorgement.

Wash green **Savoy cabbage leaves** and place them in the fridge. Just before you use them, roll out the leaves with a rolling pin and shape them to your breast shape. Cover all of the engorged area with the leaves but be careful not to put them on broken skin (place around the nipples if they are sore). Leave on for a maximum of 20 minutes until the leaves wilt. Don't leave them on for longer as this may actually reduce the milk supply.

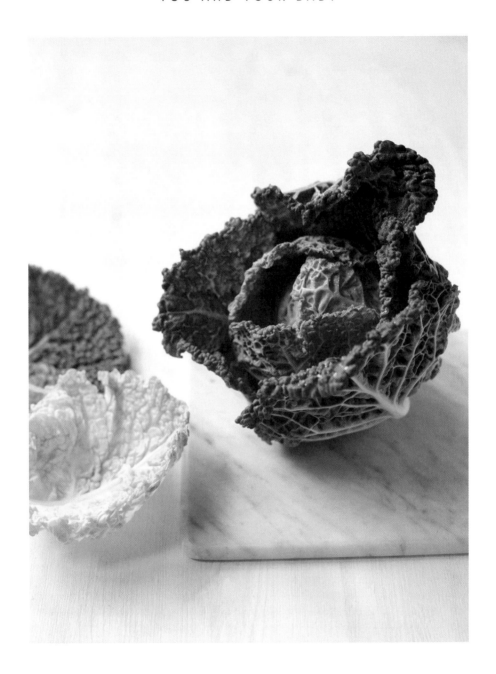

Mindful feeding

Feeding your baby can be the perfect time to slow down, to hit the pause button, and to soak up those precious moments in the magical first weeks as a mother. This moment right now, right here, is all that matters.

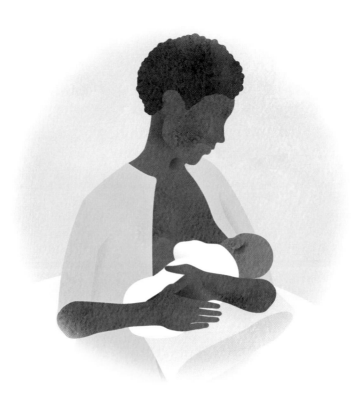

1

If you are preparing a bottle, take a moment to become present as you wait for the water to heat. If using formula, purposefully count out the scoops.

2

Turn off the television, put your phone away, and practise being present without any distractions as you feed your baby. Keep your eyes open, softly gazing at your baby. Get yourself and your baby comfortable and take a few moments to really connect with your baby. Tell him what you're doing so he can hear your voice.

3

Bring your awareness to your breathing. Notice where your back connects with the chair or your feet connect with the floor. Pay attention to the way your baby feels in your arms – that wonderful feeling of connection and protection. Notice the delicious smell of your baby and his excited anticipation of being fed in your arms. Take a few deep breaths, then resume your normal breathing as your baby begins to feed.

4

Notice how your body feels – maybe there are areas that feel tight and areas that feel soft. Just notice them. Bring your awareness to those areas. Your body is such a great source of wisdom when you pay attention to it and listen to the signals that it is giving to you.

5

Bring your attention back to your breath. As your baby finishes feeding, give gratitude for these moments with your newborn.

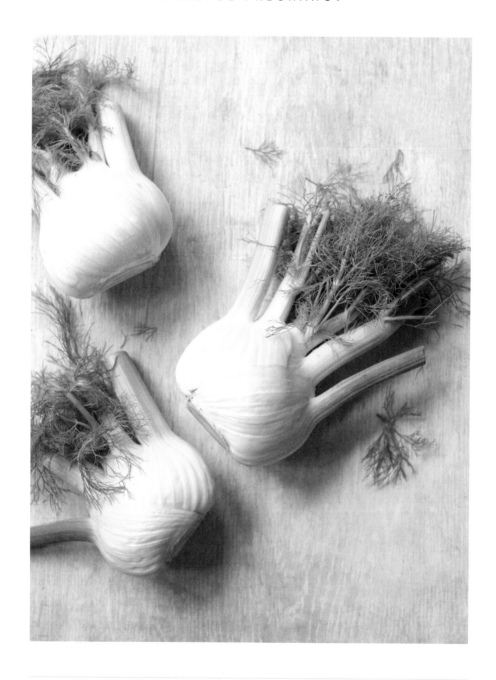

Herbal remedies for milk supply

It is very common for new mums to worry about making enough milk for their baby, so since time began many cultures have used traditional remedies to help support an abundant milk supply.

Lifestyle and stress can impact milk production, so before taking herbs or medication check that you are hydrated, eating well *(see p198)*, and resting enough. Also check your baby is latching on properly. **Fenugreek** is one of the best-known herbs to increase milk supply, but it is not recommended if you are diabetic, have a peanut allergy, or if you or your baby experience digestive upset. **Blessed thistle** is often combined with fenugreek and is found in many nursing teas. **Fennel** also supports the letdown reflex and is available in its vegetable form or as a herbal tea, although note too much can reduce milk supply, so have a maximum of three cups of fennel tea a day.

"Mindfully explore your baby's tiny fingers and toes as you feed."

Be with your baby

The focus of this meditation is to simply be present with your baby – doing nothing else but being present. Try doing this exercise when your baby is fed and calm so you can both enjoy the moment.

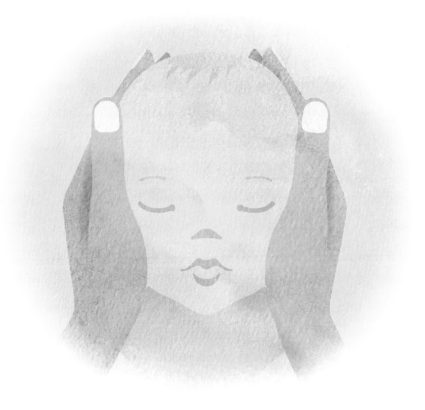

"Immerse yourself in your baby, imagining this is the very first time you have seen her face."

1

Make yourself comfortable. Allow your gaze to rest on your baby's face, smiling as you do so, and speaking softly to her.

2

As you settle, take a couple of deep breaths. Let go of any thoughts, and allow yourself to be fully present with your baby in the moment.

3

Notice your baby's perfect eyes and tiny eyelashes. Notice her tiny nose and pink cheeks, as if you're seeing all of this for the first time.

4

Notice your baby's breathing, seeing how sweet and effortless it is. Be aware of any sounds she is making.

5

Thoughts and feelings may come and go. Acknowledge them, then bring your attention back to the sounds of your baby. Focus on how you and your baby are connected forever, and by taking these few moments, you are giving her the wonderful gift of being totally present.

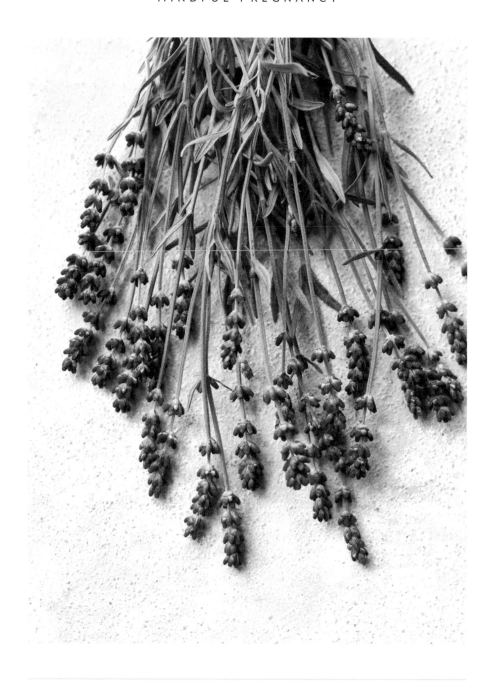

Herbal teas for insomnia

Sleep is critically important for your physical recovery and emotional wellbeing as you settle into motherhood. Chamomile and lavender make excellent herbal teas to help with relaxation and improved sleep.

One study of new mothers with poor sleep quality found that those who drank **chamomile tea** daily over two weeks reported improved sleep. To make your own tea, place four to six organic **chamomile flowers** or **buds** in a tea ball and let it steep in 250ml of just-boiled water for three to five minutes. You can also add turmeric, ginger, or honey if you prefer it spiced or sweeter. **Lavender tea** is a wonderful calming alternative. Place one teaspoon of dried organic English **lavender flowers** in a tea ball and leave to steep as above.

"If these herbal teas are new to you, try them early in the evening to see how the herbs affect you."

Mindful connection

Becoming a new parent can alter your relationship with your partner. This breathing exercise will help your mind and body recreate special memories you share, letting feelings of reconnection and intimacy emerge.

1

Sit with your eyes closed and focus on your breath. Think of a special memory of your partner or the time you first met.

2

Focus on feelings of intimacy with your partner – let those memories grow as you direct your breathing into your body.

3

Breathe in and stay with that breath as it fills your lungs and your belly. Stay with those memories of ease and connection.

4

On your next breath, allow your breath to move down deep into your pelvis, reawakening a sense of aliveness and connection. Stay with your breath as you reconnect with this sacred part of your sensual self – a part of you that may have been forgotten as a new parent. Stay with these memories.

5

Slowly bring your breath back up to your belly. Breathe in reconnection with your body and with your partner.

"Allow these memories of your partner to flood your body with curiosity, appreciation, intimacy, and love."

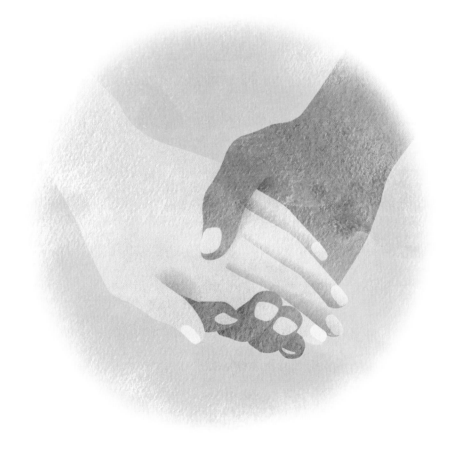

Herbal remedies for perineal healing

A daily herbal bath is a wonderfully nurturing way to help your body recover after birth. It can help reduce inflammation, shrink haemorrhoids, and promote healing of the perineum whether you had stitches or not.

To make the herbal mix you will need several muslin bags, 250g of unrefined sea salt, and 50g each of **lavender flowers**, **witch hazel flowers**, **calendula flowers**, and **chamomile flowers** (all can be purchased online). Combine all the ingredients and fill the muslin bags. Place one bag into a hot bath and allow the flowers and oils to steep in the water (your bathroom will smell divine too!). Once the bath has cooled to a comfortable temperature you can enjoy.

Another option for perineal healing is to use padsicles. These are maternity pads you presoak with **alcohol-free witch hazel** and store in the freezer to use for postpartum recovery. You can also add a drop of **lavender essential oil** or **aloe vera** if you wish. Leave to thaw for a few minutes, then apply to the perineum to reduce pain and swelling.

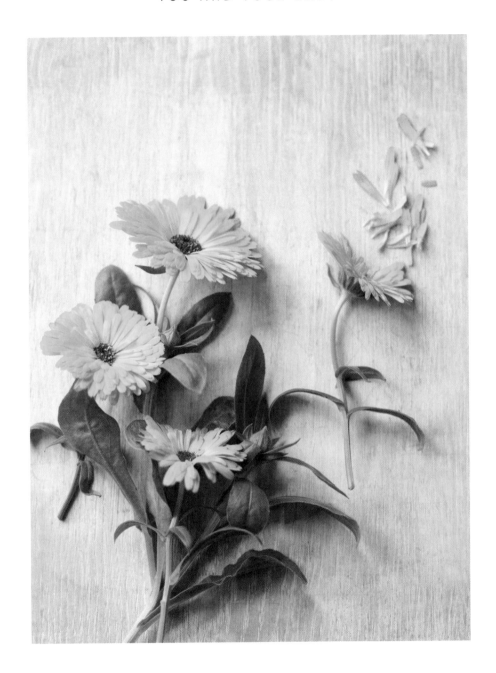

Practice and posture

As a new mum, it is recommended that you don't return to exercise for the first six weeks post-birth. However, some gentle stretching of the neck and shoulders can feel wonderful when you are carrying a newborn all day.

Early on, exercise may be the last thing on your sleep-deprived mind, but pausing for a moment of yoga when the opportunity arises allows you to create a consistent space to connect with your body and breath in this time of huge change. You can do some of the poses with your baby next to you, and you can do neck rolls while sitting upright feeding your baby. Before you return to a regular yoga practice your midwife, yoga teacher, or GP should check your core abdominal muscles for separation. Remember that your body may feel very different, so approach this new you with an attitude of acceptance.

"This is a time to generously replenish and nourish your body – physically and emotionally."

10-MINUTE SEQUENCE

A slow and gentle introduction to exercise is key after having a baby. At first you may want to just do one of these poses, depending on how you're feeling. As you get stronger and have more energy you can add a couple of poses to make a sequence.

01

NECK ROLLS

When getting to grips with different breastfeeding positions this simple exercise can relieve tension in the top of the spine and neck. Settle into Easy Pose *(see p153)*. As you exhale, let your left ear drop to your left shoulder. Pull your shoulders down. As you inhale, move your head back to neutral, then drop your chin to your chest. Repeat on the other side. Continue for a few minutes.

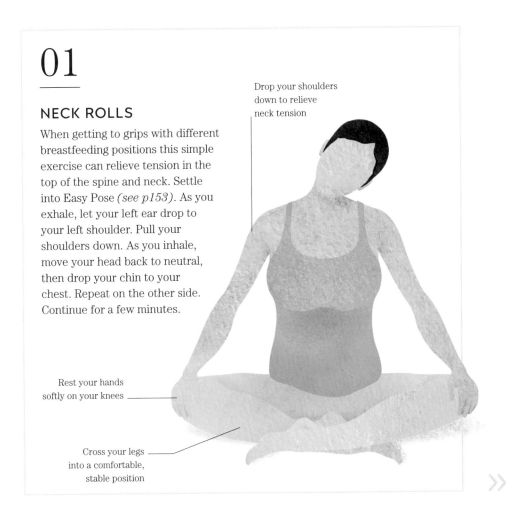

Drop your shoulders down to relieve neck tension

Rest your hands softly on your knees

Cross your legs into a comfortable, stable position

02

SEATED SIDE STRETCH

This pose emphasizes spaciousness in the upper body, which can be invigorating after feeding and carrying your newborn. Sit tall in Easy Pose, either cross-legged or with the soles of your feet together. Slowly lean over to the left so your elbow drops to the floor. Let your right arm float up but without hunching your shoulder. Breathe into the stretch for about 30 seconds, then repeat on the other side. Continue for a few minutes.

PREGNANCY HORMONES

Be mindful that your body is still under the influence of the hormone relaxin, so only use slow, gentle movements.

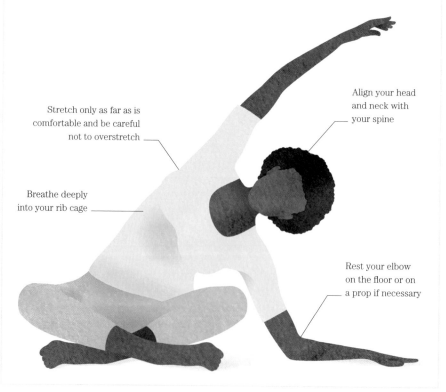

Stretch only as far as is comfortable and be careful not to overstretch

Breathe deeply into your rib cage

Align your head and neck with your spine

Rest your elbow on the floor or on a prop if necessary

03

WARRIOR POSE

As your energy returns, this power pose embodies strength, stability, and balance. Stand up slowly and move into Mountain Pose *(see p143)*. Move your feet wide apart, then turn your left foot out 90 degrees. Turn your upper body to follow the direction of your toes, inhale, and lift your arms. Exhale and bend your left knee. Lift your chin and hold for 20 seconds. Inhale, straighten your knee, turn your body forward to return to Mountain Pose, and repeat on the other side. Continue for a few minutes.

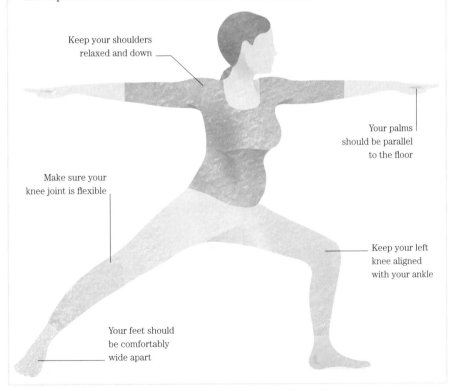

Keep your shoulders relaxed and down

Your palms should be parallel to the floor

Make sure your knee joint is flexible

Keep your left knee aligned with your ankle

Your feet should be comfortably wide apart

References

014–015 Meditation

L. Duncan et al., "Benefits Of Preparing For Childbirth With Mindfulness Training: A Randomized Controlled Trial With Active Comparison", *BMC Pregnancy and Childbirth* 17 (2017).

K. Shreffler et al., "Effect Of A Mindfulness-based Pilot Intervention On Maternal-fetal Bonding", *International Journal of Women's Health* 11 (2019), pp377–380.

I. Nyklíček et al., "Mindfulness Skills During Pregnancy: Prospective Associations With Mother's Mood And Neonatal Birth Weight", *Journal of Psychosomatic Research* 107 (2018), pp14–19.

K. Bassam et al., "Mindfulness-based Stress Reduction for Healthy Individuals: A Meta-analysis", *Journal of Psychosomatic Research* 78, no. 6 (2015), pp519–528.

W. Sriboonpimsuay et al., "Meditation for preterm birth prevention: a randomized controlled trial in Udonthani, Thailand", *International Journal of Public Health Research* 1, no. 1 (2011), pp31–39.

J. Ong et al., "A Randomized Controlled Trial Of Mindfulness Meditation For Chronic Insomnia: Effects On Daytime Symptoms And Cognitive-Emotional Arousal", *Mindfulness* 9 (2018).

022–023 Natural Remedies

M. Beckmann and O. Stock, "Antenatal Perineal Massage For Reducing Perineal Trauma", *Cochrane Database of Systematic Reviews* (2013).

026–029 Nutrition

R. Bailey et al., "Estimation Of Total Usual Dietary Intakes Of Pregnant Women In The United States", *JAMA Network Open* 2 (2019).

L. Nichols, *Real Food For Pregnancy: The Science and Wisdom of Optimal Prenatal Nutrition,* Lily Nichols, USA, 2018.

NICE, "Quality Statement 1: Healthy Eating In Pregnancy", *NICE* [web article], 2015, https://www.nice.org.uk/guidance/qs98/chapter/Quality-statement-1-Healthy-eating-in-pregnancy (accessed Feb–Jun 2019).

NHS, "Foods to Avoid in pregnancy", *NHS* [web article], Jan 2017, www.nhs.uk/conditions/pregnancy-and-baby/foods-to-avoid-pregnant (accessed Feb–Jun 2019).

030–031 Hypnobirthing

D. Spiegel, "The Mind Prepared: Hypnosis in Surgery", *Journal of the National Cancer Institute* 99, no. 17 (2007), pp1280–1281.

D. Patterson and P. Jensen "Hypnosis and clinical pain", *Psychological Bulletin* 129 (2003), pp495–521.

P. La Marca-Ghaemmaghami et al., "Second-trimester amniotic fluid corticotropin-releasing hormone and urocortin in relation to maternal stress and fetal growth in human pregnancy", *Stress* (2017).

J. Richardson et al., "Hypnosis for nausea and vomiting in cancer chemotherapy: a systematic review of the research evidence", *European Journal of Cancer Care* 16 (2007), pp402–412.

052–053 Ginger for nausea

RCOG, "The Management of Nausea and Vomiting of Pregnancy and Hyperemesis Gravidarum", *RCOG* [web article], Jun 2016, https://www.rcog.org.uk/globalassets/documents/guidelines/green-top-guidelines/gtg69-hyperemesis.pdf (accessed Feb–Jun 2019).

062–063 Vitamin D

Dovnik and F. Mujezinović, "The Association Of Vitamin D Levels With Common Pregnancy Complications", *Nutrients* 10 (2018).

NHS, "How To Get Vitamin D From Sunlight", *NHS* [web article], Aug 2018, www.nhs.uk/live-well/healthy-body/how-to-get-vitamin-d-from-sunlight (accessed Feb–Jun 2019).

084–085 Mindful eating

J. Matthews et al., "Psychosocial Predictors Of Gestational Weight Gain And The Role Of Mindfulness", *Midwifery* 56 (2018).

136–137 Medjool dates

M. Nasiri et al., "Effects Of Consuming Date Fruits (Phoenix Dactylifera Linn) On Gestation, Labor, And Delivery: An Updated Systematic Review And Meta-Analysis Of Clinical Trials", *Complementary Therapies in Medicine* 45 (2019).

168–169 Essential oils for labour

K. Najmabadi, "Systematic Review And Meta-Analysis Of Randomized Clinical Trials On The Effect Of Aromatherapy With Lavender On Labor Pain Relief", *Journal of Women's Health Care* 06 (2017).

208–209 Herbal teas for insomnia

S. Chen and C. Chen, "Effects Of Lavender Tea On Fatigue, Depression, And Maternal-Infant Attachment In Sleep-Disturbed Postnatal Women", *Worldviews on Evidence-Based Nursing* 12 (2015).

S. Chen and C. Chen, "Effects Of An Intervention With Drinking Chamomile Tea On Sleep Quality And Depression In Sleep Disturbed Postnatal Women: A Randomized Controlled Trial", *Journal of Advanced Nursing* 72 (2015).

Other suggested reading

L. Hicks et al., "Mindfulness Moderates Depression And Quality Of Prenatal Attachment In Expectant Parents", *Mindfulness* 9 (2018).

G. Kappen et al., "On The Association Between Mindfulness And Romantic Relationship Satisfaction: The Role Of Partner Acceptance", *Mindfulness* 9 (2018).

Index

ABOUT THE AUTHOR

Tracy Donegan RM is a medically trained midwife, published author, and positive birth expert. Born in Ireland, Tracy has lived and worked on three continents and currently lives in California with her husband and two sons. She is the founder and President of GentleBirth, which combines brain science, birth science, and technology, to empower parents to experience positive birth through preparation. GentleBirth is a global leader in childbirth education, with certified instructors who hail from more than a dozen countries and a mobile app available in 155 countries. The app provides guided visualizations, meditations, and breathing techniques to help prepare for a mindful birth. Tracy is a popular guest speaker, representing GentleBirth at conferences around the world and is at the forefront of the global positive birth movement.

ACKNOWLEDGMENTS

From the Author Writing a book is a lot like labour – except the sleepless nights come before the baby. It's a rollercoaster of excitement and anxiety before the final surreal moment of euphoria and disbelief when it's all over. I'm eternally grateful to my husband Philip and my two boys Cooper and Jack, who encouraged me each step of the way and gave me a wide berth, especially in the final 'trimester'. To my parents, who continue to have unwavering faith that I can do anything I set my mind to (and they've been right so far), thank you. Thank you to Claire Wedderburn-Maxwell for your editorial help and patience as we bounced ideas from both sides of the Atlantic. Thank you to Dawn Henderson and everyone at DK who believed in the importance of this book to inspire expectant mums to experience a new approach to pregnancy. Finally, sincere thanks to Mary Tighe, Joanne Bohigian, Julie Dubriollet, Ann Grauer, and Cass McNamara for generously sharing your insights and expertise before, during, and after the birth of *Mindful Pregnancy.*

From the Publisher DK would like to thank Jane Ellis for proofreading and Hilary Bird for indexing.

DISCLAIMER